CHALLENGES IN ELDER CARE

Edited by **Edward T. Zawada Jr.**

Challenges in Elder Care
http://dx.doi.org/10.5772/61984
Edited by Edward T. Zawada Jr.

Contributors

Inderpal Singh, Bilge Sözen Şahne, Stanislaw P. Stawicki, Marissa Cohen, Alaa-Eldin Mira, Ric Baxter, Elisabeth Paul, John David Nuschke, Ana Castellanos, Bruce Bartlow, Thiruvoipati Nandakumar, Edward T. Zawada, Jr.

Published by InTech

Janeza Trdine 9, 51000 Rijeka, Croatia

Publishing Process Manager Andrea Koric
Technical Editor SPi Global
Cover InTech Design team

First published September, 2016
Printed in Croatia

Additional hard copies can be obtained from orders@intechopen.com

Challenges in Elder Care, Edited by Edward T. Zawada Jr.
p. cm.
Print ISBN 978-953-51-2664-5
Online ISBN 978-953-51-2665-2

For EU product safety concerns:
IN TECH d.o.o., Prolaz Marije Krucifikse Kozulić 3, 51000 Rijeka, Croatia,
info@intechopen.com or visit our website at intechopen.com.

Meet the editor

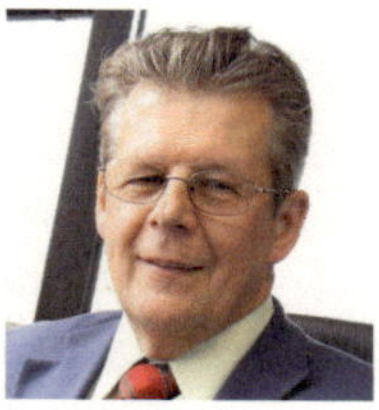

Edward T. Zawada Jr., MD, was born in Chicago, Illinois, in 1947. He graduated with a Bachelor of Science degree *summa cum laude* from Loyola University Chicago in 1969 and an MD degree *summa cum laude* from the Loyola Stritch School of Medicine in 1973. He was inducted into *Alpha Omega Alpha* in 1972. He trained in internal medicine and nephrology in David Geffen School of Medicine at UCLA where he later served as an assistant professor of medicine. He had a long career in academic medicine at the University of Utah, Medical College of Virginia, and Sanford School of Medicine of the University of South Dakota where he is a professor and chairman emeritus of the Department of Internal Medicine. He is board certified by the American Board of Internal Medicine in internal medicine, nephrology, geriatrics, and critical care medicine. He also has board certifications in nutrition by the American College of Nutrition, pharmacology by the American Society of Clinical Pharmacology, and hypertension by the American Society of Hypertension. He has been awarded with a fellowship status by the American College of Physicians, the American College of Chest Physicians, the American Heart Association, the American Society of Nephrology, the American Geriatrics Society, the American College of Clinical Pharmacology, the Society for Vascular Medicine, and the Society of Critical Care Medicine. He was awarded a distinguished service award by the South Dakota Medical Society in 2002 for a career devoted to medical education and master of the American College of Physicians in 2005.

Contents

Preface

This collection is an update on caring for geriatric patients, often defined as those over 65 years of age, which has seen an increased demand for expertise since the first baby boomers reached this milestone approximately 5 years ago. Patients over 80 years old (oldest old) are the most rapidly growing segment of our society, which is likely to continue for another 18 years as the boomers continue to advance through their 70s into their 80s.

The first chapter recalls some of the newer and very severe diseases and health problems facing them today. The second chapter reviews the concept of frailty. A famous quote of Thomas Hobbes reminds us that we will all reach a point in our lives in which we experience the fact that "Life is nasty, brutish, and short" as we become weaker, lose mobility, have impaired vision and hearing, develop chronic pain, and lose mental acuity. Elder care differs from other segments of the population due to altered pathophysiology due to aging. Homeostasis becomes homeostenosis. Diagnosis and treatment of the elderly take longer, require multidisciplinary expertise, and must integrate the known longitudinal features of diseases with the altered pathophysiology. The tool of geriatric assessment to accomplish this is described in an additional chapter. Prescription of medications for health problems in the elderly requires consideration of altered dosing schedules and care to avoid drug-drug interactions with those medications prescribed by other healthcare providers. This topic is covered in the chapter on polypharmacy. In caring for the elderly, our first choice should be medication reduction or "MED RED." If we do start new medications, we should "start low and go slow." We must adjust the dose for reduced renal and hepatic function. Elders are often not cured of their diseases, just managed to the point of restoring functional status. They have chronic illnesses and even chronic critical illnesses but live on. The rise of the long-term acute care hospital has occurred to combine management of serious illness with a rehabilitation process to return the patient as much as possible to independent activities of daily living. A chapter in this work deals with this novel care pathway. Finally, in today's world, patients can be kept alive for prolonged periods of time by heroic life support measures. A final chapter deals with an update on the ethics of caring for the elderly in the intensive care unit (ICU) with the most dangerous illnesses or combinations of failed organ systems called multisystem organ failure.

In conclusion, this work is an update on newer and serious clinical problems facing our expanding elderly population. Newer tools, newer locations, and newer ethics are reviewed concerning the care of the frail elderly who face the most dangerous medical problems, which most often cannot be cured. Thought must be given in their diagnosis as to how much they can tolerate the diagnostic tests, whether adding a new medication or reducing an old one is a solution to some problems, and how we avoid prolonged heroic efforts, which might be futile yet prolong suffering.

Edward T. Zawada Jr. M.D., M.A.C.P,
Professor and Chairman Emeritus
Department of Internal Medicine,
Sanford School of Medicine,
University of South Dakota, United States of America

Chapter 1

Introductory Chapter: Overview of Challenges in Geriatric Medicine in 2016

Edward T. Zawada

Additional information is available at the end of the chapter

http://dx.doi.org/10.5772/64259

Trained in nephrology from 1974 to 1976, I began to consider myself a geriatric specialist beginning in 1983 when I compiled what I believe was the first subspecialty textbook of geriatric medicine, *Geriatric Nephrology and Urology* [1]. I became board certified in geriatrics by the American Board of Internal Medicine in 1988, several years later but now nearly 30 years ago. In the 1990s, I helped to develop a Geriatric Assessment Program for Sioux Valley Medical Center in Sioux Falls, South Dakota, a MEDRED (*med*ication *red*uction) clinic program for correction of polypharmacy [2] in rural South Dakota, and published original geriatric and gerontology research. My clinical research included the identification of nutritional deficiencies of the elderly [3] and the use of biomarkers such as brain natriuretic peptide (BNP) to assist in the prevention of readmission to the hospital for elders with chronic congestive heart failure [4]. My basic science research focused on the role of dietary control of obesity to slow renal senescence [5, 6]. After 2000, I assisted in the founding and ongoing teaching effort of a Fellowship in Geriatrics. Based on my dedication to the care of the elderly verified by the above experiences, I feel justified in providing a brief summary of the most common clinical problems I face daily in the year 2016 and summarize the importance of each of the chapters in this collection to geriatric medicine from my perspective.

The most frustrating clinical problems I now frequently face in caring for elders include intracranial bleeds due to falls in elders on new anticoagulants for atrial fibrillation, severe hypoxemia in elders with pneumonia, recurrent advanced congestive heart failure in those failing medical therapy, *Clostridium difficile* colitis refractory to oral antibiotics, acute renal deterioration associated with multiorgan dysfunction in patients with pneumonia or heart failure, morbid obesity resulting in pulmonary and hepatic dysfunction, and myelodysplasia resulting in refractory pancytopenia. I give a brief explanation of the difficulty in managing these problems and their relevance to chapters in this book.

Devastating neurologic diseases that are common in the elderly include dementia and stroke, which are difficult to prevent and unpredictable in occurrence. On the other hand, potentially avoidable but even more difficult to manage neurologic catastrophes for elders are the intracranial bleeds associated with falls [7]. The difficulty in controlling these bleeds is greater when patients have been receiving therapy with antiplatelet therapy or anticoagulants, especially the newer agents that are less readily reversible. Because of the high mortality of patients with this problem and possible reversibility, I devote the largest part of this introduction to details in managing this problem.

I start with a brief case which was so striking that I recall it frequently. A prominent attorney and past president of the board of our health system was reasonably fit in his mid-1980s tripped and hit his head during a strenuous morning of exercise. He had been taking clopidogrel for prior cardiac stent placement. After a brief delay, he collapsed and was in coma. He was found to have severe intracranial hemorrhage, which was refractory to an attempt at correction by transfusion of 10 units of platelets and administration of desmopressin (DDAVP) in the dose of 0.3 g/kg. Bleeding continued, and he did not survive.

The most common cause of death seen month after month as I sit in at our trauma morbidity and mortality conference is the patient receiving warfarin for atrial fibrillation who developed a subdural or other intracranial bleed after a fall. Warfarin must be reversed to lower the INR less than 1.4 in these cases with as many units of fresh-frozen plasma as needed or infusion of three- or four-factor prothrombin complex concentrate [8]. I recommend the four-factor prothrombin complex in the following doses:

If the INR is 2 to <4, give 25 units/kg; maximum of 2500 units

If the INR is 4–6, give 35 units/kg; maximum of 3500 units

If the INR is >6, give 50 units/kg; maximum of 5000 units

Recently, reversal of the factor Xa and direct thrombin inhibitors has become available [14]. Idarucizumab is now available for the reversal of dabigratan (i.e., trade name Pradaxa), the direct thrombin inhibitor. The dose should be 5 g intravenously (administered as two separate 2.5-g doses of no more than 15 min apart).

The factor Xa inhibitors include rivaroxaban (trade name, Xarelto) and epixaban (trade name, Eliquis). A reversal agent for factor Xa inhibitors is in development (andexanet alfa). It appears to act within minutes and persist for 2 h after intravenous administration of a dose of 400 (for apixaban) or 800 mg (for rivaroxaban). It may also be necessary to follow a bolus with a 2-h infusion of 4 mg/min (for apixaban) or 8 mg/min (for rivaroxaban). A review of some of the other common iatrogenic problems due to medications is presented in a chapter on "geriatric assessment" and a chapter on "polypharmacy".

Community-acquired pneumonia (CAP) has a yearly rate of disease of 5 per 1000 population and a mortality of 13.6%. Several cases that require ICU admission have mortality as high as 36% which increases even higher for each decade above 60 years of age [9, 10]. The problem is made worse by the emergence of organisms resistant to frequently used antibiotics such as methicillin-resistant *Staphylococcus aureus* or MRSA. Newer life-support techniques for managing severe hypoxia have been developed, which include pronation, extracorporeal membrane oxygenation, nitric oxide administration, and intravenous or inhaled therapy with prostaglandins. Details of each of these expensive, often invasive techniques are beyond the scope of this chapter. However, a daily question facing physicians caring for elders with severe hypoxia is whether these rescue life-support therapies should be made available to the advanced age groups. The chapter on ethics in this collection speaks about this issue.

Congestive heart failure remains one of the most common conditions requiring hospital admission. Newer strategies for prevention and management have exploded in the past 30 years. Angiotensin blockade, b-blockers, statins, very powerful diuretic combinations, newer inotropes, intraaortic balloon pumps, venoarterial extracorporeal membrane oxygenation (VA ECMO), and commercial availability of ventricular assist devices (VADs) illustrate the vast spectrum of management now available for this problem [11]. As mentioned previously, biomarkers have become increasingly useful in diagnosis and management of patients with heart failure. To distinguish cardiac from pulmonary causes of dyspnea, BNP has become an important diagnostic tool, and the test can be used in titrating the management of heart failure by repeating levels after diuresis. Other biomarkers used in managing patients with breathlessness include ST2 (an interleukin released in heart injury and stretch) and higher sensitivity troponin, which are both strong predictors of mortality. Finally, procalcitonin is used in such patients to diagnose concomitant pneumonia which requires antibiotic therapy [15, 12].

Gastroenterologic problems that I encounter the most include diverticulitis with and without bowel perforation, colon cancer requiring resection, and *C. difficile* colitis (Cdiff). The last issue may result from treating sepsis and infections associated with the first two topics and can be considered an epidemic in the geriatric segment of our society. It now stands as the most commonly reported nosocomial infection in the United States. While traditionally this infection has been an inpatient issue, it is now being recognized as a growing concern in the outpatient setting as well [13].

Some of these increased burdens are related to an epidemic strain that has been well described in the literature since the early 2000s. With regard to age, there is no group of patients that has experienced this problem with such dramatic consequences as the elderly. Those over the age of 65 years have the greatest incidence of disease as well as the greatest mortality rate. In addition, they demonstrate a higher recurrence rate, which not only contributes to a higher likelihood of death but leads to substantial morbidity and reduced quality of life. This recurrence rate is related to inadequate control of the infection due to a poor immune response with insufficient anti-toxin antibody production and inability to replenish a healthy microbiota within the colon.

This infection is diagnosed with clinical suspicion and fairly simple laboratory testing. Most patients have one or both of the dominant risk factors, which include recent contact with the health-care setting and recent use of antibacterial therapy. The dominant symptoms include diarrhea and abdominal discomfort. While the white blood cell count can be normal with this infection, it is usually elevated with more significant disease, and very high counts are not uncommon and may even point a clinician toward this diagnosis. With regard to testing, stool can be sent for a variety of assays. Enzyme immunoassay that detects toxin has been utilized for many years but has reduced sensitivity. The newer amplification tests for the toxin genes were expected to help with this issue, but they may reveal positive results in a patient colonized with *C. difficile* who has other reasons for their symptoms. Thus, clinical suspicion and pretest probability need to be adequate for testing to be ordered. Other important rules of testing include only testing liquid stool, avoiding multiple consecutive tests, avoiding repeat testing while on appropriate therapy, and avoiding a "test of cure" when symptoms have resolved.

The management of this infection has been problematic due to the limited number of therapies and the recurrent nature of the disease. Metronidazole (oral or intravenous) and oral vancomycin have been the two dominant therapies that have been utilized over the past several decades. Metronidazole is now reserved for those with mild to moderate disease, while vancomycin can be used across the spectrum, including those with severe disease. Combination therapy is not well supported by data except in the critically ill population when impaired gut motility may be a concern. Unfortunately, the recurrence rate for each of these therapies is unacceptably high, and newer therapies are needed. One of those therapies may be fidaxomicin, which has shown a lower recurrence rate in clinical trials. While there have been concerns about the cost of this drug in the past, it has been debated that the cost of the drug may be more desirable than the cost of recurrent disease. Unfortunately, clear guidance does not currently exist on this matter, and even fidaxomicin carries some risk of recurrence. Thus, alternative therapy has been utilized that centers on a principle difference than eradication of the organism. Fecal microbiota transplantation is being increasingly used in an effort to replenish healthy bacterial flora within the colon and outcompete *C. difficile*, effectively breaking the recurrent cycle of infection. This can be administered through a post-pyloric nasogastric tube, through enema, or via colonoscopy. The importance of avoiding future antibacterial therapy should be stressed if this treatment is to have lasting effects for the patient.

As this disease poses great risk to elderly patients, the dominant approach should be prevention. Unfortunately, these patients are high utilizers of the health-care system, and they are often exposed to antibacterial therapy as well as sites within the system where the organism may be acquired. Clinicians need to take great care when deciding if antibacterial therapy is truly indicated for a given condition. Common conditions that are often treated with unnecessary antibacterial therapy include upper respiratory tract infections, asymptomatic bacteriuria, and skin conditions such as stasis dermatitis. Hopefully, with appropriate antibiotic stewardship, as well as adequate infection control measures, the incidence of this disease within this vulnerable population will fall. Further assistance may come with vaccine development, and clinical trials are currently ongoing.

Advances in dialysis and renal transplantation have led to wide availability of end-stage renal failure therapy offered to people of all ages [1, 6]. The financial impact has been staggering in elderly individuals, especially considering that such life support is provided to outpatients who are not very mobile and who have outlived members of their nuclear family. Hence, the cost must also include transport to and from dialysis centers. Renal deterioration is often silent until a final snowball of metabolic crises, which create life-threatening illness and subsequent severe deconditioning. The chapter presented here on geriatric assessment deals with carefully ferreting out serious problems in stubborn, stoic elders, which might be buried by a multiplicity of other illnesses which create more symptoms.

Elders often suffer from a variety of cancers whose incidence increases with age. A particularly frustrating and not uncommon hematologic problem is the patient with refractory anemia, resistant leukopenia, and intractable thrombocytopenia. These may be the consequence of a primary cancer, a side effect of cancer chemotherapy, or due to the problem of myelofibrosis.

Primary myelofibrosis is a myeloproliferative neoplasm in which there is ineffective erythropoiesis and the bone-marrow deposition of fibrous connective tissue.

Most patients present with anemia, marked splenomegaly, early satiety, and systemic symptoms of severe fatigue, low-grade fever, night sweats, bone pain, and weight loss. Essential thrombocythemia and polycythemia vera can both undergo delayed disease transformation into a fibrotic state resulting in secondary myelofibrosis. Allogeneic hematopoietic cell transplantation is the only treatment modality with a curative potential in primary myelofibrosis for which most patients will not be a candidate. Other treatments can only be used for symptom management and will primarily consist of frequent transfusions. The patients become weaker and weaker, develop pancytopenia, and often die of sepsis. Ethics again plays a role in deciding how far to go with cancers and myelofibrosis, especially since treatments for cancers are often poorly tolerated, and adding advanced life support to sustain their lives for more of such therapy becomes a difficult decision for families and physicians more so than patients who will frequently request a transition to palliation or comfort care.

Morbid obesity management has become a science of its own—bariatrics. The year 2016 commonly results in a requirement for two skill sets in clinical medicine, bariatrics, and geriatrics. The bariatric geriatric patient is more susceptible to multisystem organ failure and requires different pharmacology, different medical devices, and different nutritional management of the frequent failure of lungs, heart, liver, and kidneys in these patients. These patients frequently develop sleep apnea, edema, skin infections and ulcers, diabetes, impaired mobility, hypertension, thromboembolism, pulmonary hypertension, cor pulmonale, and renal insufficiency. Pharmacokinetics of medication administration and nutrition during illness are complicated and confusing as to whether to base them on actual or ideal weight. When hospitalized, they require specialized beds, wheelchairs, and extra staff for assisted transfers at an increased cost. Special scans (computerized tomography (CT) and magnetic resonance imaging (MRI)) are often delayed or denied because of physical constraints of the scanner opening and weight limits on the imaging tables. There is a chapter in this collection on frailty in the elderly. The obese elder is frail but will not be recognized for this impairment because of the stereotype that a small thin person is frail.

In the past 20 years, there has been a new component to the health-care continuum, the long-term, acute-care unit (LTAC). Elders and even younger patients often have a lesser set of physiologic disturbances after hospital or ICU discharge but which persist for weeks or months. They require additional time for healing, for resumption of activities of daily life, and instrumental activities of daily life. They often require weeks of ongoing treatments for the reason for hospitalization such as antibiotics for infections, wound management requiring ongoing debridement, enteral or parenteral nutrition, continued ventilator support by tracheostomy, and even dialysis. They require additional physical therapy, speech therapy, and occupational therapy to resume independent functional status. One of the chapters in this collection describes the growth of this new additional component of the health-care continuum: home, primary care, hospital, ICU, back to the hospital, long-term acute care, skilled nursing facility, and then back home.

In summary, this introductory chapter points to the direction for those which follow. The clinical problems I have described are often better diagnosed in a single visit by the tool of Geriatric Assessment. The above problems require complicated medication combinations, which require knowledge of pitfalls in initial boluses and maintenance dosing in the elderly as covered in a chapter to follow. The lack of cardiac reserve in complicated illnesses in the elderly can be monitored by biomarkers. The ethical dilemmas we face in the care of the most seriously ill elders with problems such as the above have led to an exponential growth in techniques of palliative care and hospice care including the legalization of physician-assisted suicide. Several chapters will deal with these moral, philosophical, and ethical issues. The principles of managing patients over 60 have resulted in the creation of a field of clinical specialists who can become board certified in Geriatrics. The anatomy, physiology, demographics, and social issues of aging have likewise expanded a body of knowledge, which has been identified as gerontology. This publication seeks to summarize several of the more common clinical problems and their management which have come to the fore in the care of elders in 2016.

Author details

Edward T. Zawada

Address all correspondence to: ezawada@sio.midco.net

Sanford School of Medicine, University of South Dakota, Sioux Falls, South Dakota

References

[1] Zawada ET, Sica DA, editors: Geriatric Nephrology and Urology, Wright PSG publisher, Littleton, Massachussetts, pp 558, 1985.

[2] Schrader SL, Dressing B, Zawada ET Jr, Blue R: The medication reduction projects: combating polypharmacy in South Dakota elders through community-based interventions. South Dakota Journal of Medicine 1996; 49(12):441–448.

[3] Schrader SL, Schrank M, Blue R, Zawada ET Jr, Trujillo AL: Meal-Mate: improving the nutritional status of elders using a milk-based nutritional supplement. South Dakota Journal of Medicine 1995; 48:301–311.

[4] Zawada ET Jr: Principal Investigator, Multidisciplinary care clinic to reduce morbidity due to congestive heart failure in the elderly. Sanford Research Institute, July 12, 2000-June 30, 2002.

[5] Alavi FK, Zawada ET Jr, Simmons H: Renal hemodynamic and histological consequences of a diet high in fat, protein, or sucrose in obese Zucker rates. Clinical Nephrology 1995; 43:122–130.

[6] Zawada ET Jr: The aging kidney, in Textbook of Nephrology, Massryl S and Glassock R., editors, Williams and Wilkins publishers, Baltimore, Maryland, 1989, 2nd edition, Chapter 58, pp 996–1002.

[7] Bullock MR, Chestnut R, Ghajer J et al: Surgical management of acute subdural hematoma. Neurosurgery 2006; 58(3 suppl.):S25–S46.

[8] Meyer SA, Rincon R: Treatment of intracerebral hemorrhage. Lancet Neurology 2005; 4:662–672.

[9] Fine MJ, Smith MA, Carson CA, et al: Prognosis and outcomes of patients with community-acquired pneumonia, a meta analysis. JAMA 1996; 275:134–141.

[10] Reed MJ, Siddiqui A, Keshava K, Sl-Asad M, Foltzer M: Specific infections with critical care implications. In Comprehensive Critical Care: Adult. Pamela Roberts and Rob Todd, editors. Society of Critical Care Medicine publisher. Mount Prospect, Illinois, 2012, pp 491–510.

[11] Gayat E, Mebazza A: Severe heart failure, cardiogenic shock, and pericardial tamponade. In, Comprehensive Critical Care: Adult. Pamela R. Roberts and S. Robb, editors. Society of Critical Care Medicine, publisher. Mount Prospect, Illinois, 2012; pp 153–166.

[12] Wettersten N, Maisel AS: Biomarkers for heart failure: an update for practitioners of internal medicine. American Journal of Medicine 2016; 129:560–567.

[13] Interview with Matt Miles MD. Infectious Disease Consultant, Redding, California, March 14, 2016.

[14] Connors JM: Antidote for factor Xa anticoagulants. New England Journal of Medicine 2015; 373:2471-2472.

[15] Tefferi A: Management of primary myelofibrosis. UpToDate. 2016.

Chapter 2

Patient Frailty: Key Considerations, Definitions and Practical Implications

Marissa S. Cohen, Elisabeth Paul,
John David Nuschke, Julia C. Tolentino,
Ana V. Castellanos Mendez, Alaa-Eldin A. Mira,
Ric A. Baxter and Stanislaw P. Stawicki

Additional information is available at the end of the chapter

http://dx.doi.org/10.5772/64296

Abstract

By 2020, the elderly (≥65-year-old) world population is projected to exceed one billion individuals. This demographic megatrend has brought topics such as physiological age and frailty to the forefront of medical research efforts around the globe. The concept of frailty has evolved significantly since the mid-twentieth century. The outdated stereotype of a "thin, stooped, slow octogenarian" has transitioned to a more scientific and objective understanding of the problem. Still, a comprehensive and concise definition of "frailty" remains elusive. Until such a definition is firmly established and universally agreed upon, clinicians continue to rely on the somewhat subjective conceptual framework of today. In this chapter, the authors review key issues pertaining to clinical management of frail patients, including diagnosis/identification, preventive strategies, therapeutic approaches, and common pitfalls. The relationship between frailty, various domains of life, and functional status is also discussed. Finally, we will touch upon the concepts of end-of-life and goals of care, focusing on their relationship to frailty.

Keywords: Frailty, Chronological age, Physiological age, Aging process, Objective assessment

1. Introduction

The world population is projected to exceed 7.5 billion in 2020, with one billion to reach or exceed 65 years of age [1, 2]. This demographic change has made frailty the focus of considerable scientific research, generating increasing interest during the past two decades [3–5]. As more people make the transition across the life span [6], better understanding of the corresponding changes and considerations is required. The concept of frailty has evolved substantially over the past five decades. The stereotypical description of a "thin, stooped, slow octogenarian" [7], although very vivid and generally reflective of a frail patient, has not been matched with an equally concise definition. A comprehensive and objective definition of frailty is needed in order to effectively diagnose, research, and improve the understanding of this condition. Until such definition is universally agreed upon, clinicians will have to do their best diagnosing frailty within the currently established framework. This chapter reviews some of the key issues that practitioners may encounter when treating frail patients, including its identification, preventive, and therapeutic options, as well as common pitfalls. We also discuss the relationship between frailty and various domains of life and functional status, with a brief overview of recent trends in the area of goals of care and end-of-life considerations.

2. What is frailty?

Frailty is a multifactorial phenomenon (**Figure 1**) that affects multiple domains of life (**Table 1**). Our understanding of frailty has advanced significantly since the late 1960s, when frail patients were described as "...confused, restless, incontinent... [and] ...old" [8]. Twenty years later, the frail population was described as "...elderly people with multiple problems..." [9]. Today's definitions are more dynamic, elegant, and refined, with two main models of frailty dominating the recent literature [10, 11]. The "phenotype model" of frailty, described as "...a biologic syndrome of decreased reserve and impaired resistance to stressors, resulting from cumulative declines across multiple physiological systems, and causing vulnerability to

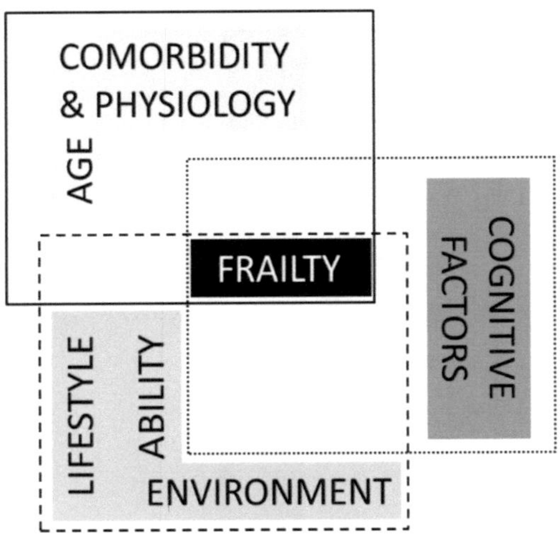

Figure 1. Venn diagram showing the overlap of different domains, all of which contribute to the eventual development and progression of frailty.

http://dx.doi.org/10.5772/64296

adverse outcomes…" was proposed by Fried et al. [12]. This model requires the presence of three out of the following five phenotypic criteria in order to define frailty: (a) low grip strength; (b) low/decreased energy levels; (c) slow walking speed; (d) low physical activity; and/or (e) unintentional weight loss [12]. The second model, developed by Rockwood et al. takes into account "assets" and "deficits" which either aid or are detrimental to a patient's independent functioning [13, 14]. This model is closely tied to various indices currently used as tools for assessing the degree of frailty in patients.

Impairment	Activities affected	Risks
Ambulatory dysfunction	Driving	Elder abuse/neglect
Cognitive decline	Social interaction	Financial theft
Impaired judgment	General functional level	Depression
Medication side effects	Access to services/care	Suicide
Impairment in eyesight		Lack of understanding
Impairment in hearing		
Education/prevention		
Holistic assessment of the individual	Realistic discussions about specific risks	
Shared decision-making	Advance directive	
Established power-of-attorney	Durable power of attorney	
Do not wait for a crisis	Review of medication profile	
Screening for depression		
Resources		
Family and immediate social network	Faith community	
Adult day care communities	Area association on aging	
Alzheimer's association	Palliative care programs	
Home health programs		

Compiled with permission from Keller et al. (1999). *J Am Geriatr Soc* 47(11):1319–25; McGadney BF. (1995) *African American Research Perspectives* 2(1):34; Panza et al. (2010). *Am J Geriatr Psychiatry* 18(2):98–116; Schulman-Green et al. (2006). *Patient Education & Counseling* 63(1):145–151; Walsh F. (2012). *Annual Review of Gerontology & Geriatrics* 32(1):151–172.

Table 1. Conditions that may lead to the development of frailty while also placing the individuals at various types of associated risk. An outline of educational and community resources is provided as well.

Boers et al. [15] argue that the existing definitions of frailty are limited because the word "syndrome" should be reserved for defining phenotype characteristics that constitute a set of symptoms and signs representing a health condition. They also argue that the classic World Health Organization definition of health is outdated and that a new, more dynamic concept of health as "…the resilience or capacity to cope, and to maintain and restore one's integrity, equilibrium, and sense of well-being in three domains: physical, mental, and social…" opens the door to simply defining frailty as "the weakening of health" [15–17]. Currently, there is insufficient evidence to accept a single definition of frailty [14], and the ongoing debate highlights the need for a consensus [18].

Using the definition of frailty as a "...decreased reserve and resistance to stressors..." [19] highlights the importance of individualized, careful approach when weighing risks and benefits of various interventions [20–22]. In this context, an "intervention" could range from an elective surgical procedure to initial administration of an oral hypoglycemic agent in a diabetic patient. For example, one prospective study found that patients deemed as "intermediately frail" or "frail" were more likely to experience postoperative complications [23]. Some authors suggest that frailty should be routinely measured as part of the perioperative patient risk assessment in older individuals, pointing out that most current surgical risk scores do not adequately take frailty into consideration [24]. In one study, patients deemed fit by Comprehensive Geriatric Assessment (CGA [25]) with diffuse large-cell lymphoma had better survival and chemotherapy response rates when compared to their "more frail" counterparts [26]. One systematic review suggested that more than half of older cancer patients in the United Kingdom were "pre-frail" or "frail", and identified that these groups were at increased risk of all-cause mortality, chemotherapy intolerance, and postoperative complications [27, 28]. Frailty may also compound the problem of pre-existing medical conditions, mainly via multiple "feedback" mechanisms, where frailty facilitates the downward clinical spiral [29]. For example, recurrent episodes of hypoglycemia may occur unnoticed due to the impaired autonomic response in the frail, elderly diabetic patient. This, in turn, may result in repeated subclinical central nervous system insults, which may lead to worsening cognitive dysfunction (e.g., progressive dementia) and physical frailty [29]. Frailty may also be associated with greater incidence of cardiovascular death, myocardial infarction, and stroke [30]. Taken together, the above examples may be applicable across various clinical settings where disease, treatment, and frailty dynamically interact [31, 32]. Evidence also shows that although patients considered "pre-frail" and "frail" had greater morbidity and mortality when compared to their "robust" counterparts, the median age in the three frailty groups was similar, supporting the notion that both chronological *and* physiological age play a role in the "frailty equation" [30, 33].

Frailty is also an independent predictor of falls, delirium, disability, and hospitalization [34]. Better understanding of frailty, coupled with the ability to identify it, is critical to our ability to control, and possibly modulate, associated physiological and cognitive changes. This not only has significant implications for patients and their quality of life but also presents an opportunity to reduce health care-associated costs of frailty by focusing on effective preventive strategies [35–37]. Despite the growing focus around frailty, screening and risk stratification are still limited, the CGA is underutilized, and the involvement of geriatric specialists is far from routine [38]. In summary, there is need for better identification of frail patients in order to optimize their clinical management and adequately counsel patients regarding risks and benefits of any proposed treatments [39].

3. Frailty: identification and assessment

The gold standard for identifying frail individuals is the Comprehensive Geriatric Assessment (CGA) [40]. The CGA requires a team of doctors, nurses, and therapists to jointly establish a patient's matrix of bio-psycho-social needs [41, 42]. In studies, CGA has been closely associated with the Canadian Study of Health and Aging (CSHA) frailty index [43, 44]. Due to the amount of effort required to complete a CGA for all at-risk patients, it is challenging for the non-geriatric practitioner to effectively mobilize the required resources. Consequently, extensive research has been performed to find a simpler method of identifying and quantifying frailty.

Another model outlines a phenotypic definition of frailty [12, 45]. This model, proposed by Fried, is relatively simple and requires little modification to the routine, standard-of-care medical practice when collecting and assessing required variables. However, its translation into clinical practice may be challenging [40]. Critics of Fried's definition argue that it does not sufficiently address cognitive aspects of frailty. Some propose that adding a mini mental state exam (MMSE) and the Isaacs Set test may improve the predictive validity of the combined screening tests [46]. It has been shown that targeted questionnaires can be very effective in evaluating frailty in the elderly population, especially when looking at aspects of "psycho-physical state" and frailty [47]. Such questionnaires may be useful in identifying and quantifying various cognitive and mood aspects of frailty.

One systematic review showed that the most sensitive screening tools used to measure frailty are gait speed <0.8 m/s, timed-up-and-go-test of >10 s, and the PRISMA 7 score of ≥3 [48]. These criteria had sensitivities of 0.99, 0.93, and 0.83 and specificities of 0.64, 0.62, and 0.83, respectively [48]. Of importance, most of the research on screening tools originates from the outpatient setting, with relatively less experience regarding screening for frailty in the hospital [49]. In summary, if a CGA is unavailable, the practitioner should utilize multi-modality, phenotype-based approaches that incorporate multiple, complementary screening tools outlined above.

4. Frailty versus comorbidities: similar but different

The concept of frailty rests on the idea that declining physiological reserve and function leads to susceptibility toward adverse outcomes and poor resolution of acute medical events and injuries [40]. At this point, it is important to discuss the relationship between frailty and comorbidity burden. Although it is intuitive that decline in physiological reserve is related to age, frailty measurements are independent of chronological age. Chronological age, frailty, and the increased prevalence of chronic health conditions are inextricably linked. Approximately 25–50% of the population >85 years of age can be characterized as being frail or vulnerable to adverse outcomes after an exposure to acute stress [40, 50, 51]. However, chronological age does not directly correlate with frailty, which is where comorbidity assessment may provide valuable quantitative insight as a co-variate.

There are several comorbidity indices, each of which offers slightly different perspective on the patient's comorbidity burden. Although a complete discussion of instruments used to quantify comorbidities is beyond the scope of this chapter, we will provide an overview of the topic. The Charlson Comorbidity Index (CCI) considers a pre-defined, weighted set of medical diagnoses and has been shown to predict healthcare resource utilization, clinical risk stratification, and mortality [52, 53]. The Elixhauser index considers variable characteristics of medical conditions across different patient populations, using a set of 30 comorbidities to predict outcomes such as length of stay, hospital charges, and mortality [54]. One Elixhauser index derivative consists of a simplified score with good utility in estimating the effect of comorbidities on clinical outcomes [55].

The Comorbidity-Polypharmacy Score (CPS) combines comorbidities and polypharmacy into a simple, yet potentially accurate measurement of frailty [33]. It is a sum of all pre-existing conditions and medications [56]. CPS weighs the "severity" of comorbidities based on the number of medications necessary to treat each respective chronic condition [33, 57]. In clinical studies, CPS correlated with morbidity, mortality, readmissions, post-emergency department (ED) triage, and the need for discharge to skilled nursing/extended care facility [33, 56–60]. CPS may thus constitute the "missing link" that uses the "intensity" of polypharmacy to connect the concepts of frailty and comorbidity.

5. Frailty: multidisciplinary and interdisciplinary approaches

Frailty is inextricably associated with several determinants of a patient's overall health status, including genetic predispositions, environmental factors, and comorbid conditions [61, 62, 40]. It naturally follows that the optimal approach to caring for frail patients is a collaborative one [63]. Consequently, treatment teams should include participants from various specialties, including generalists and specialists, smoking cessation counselors, social workers, mental health professionals, physical and occupational therapists, nutrition experts, wound care specialist, and nurses [64–68]. Major themes involved in the overall "frailty equation" are shown in **Figure 2**.

A collaborative approach to identification, prevention, and management of frailty can be facilitated by establishing areas of subspecialty within existing medical disciplines that focus on the care of the elderly and the frail [69, 70]. For example, during exploratory work on the concept of geriatric surgery, it was emphasized that this new surgical subspecialty should have multidisciplinary character [71]. Among other recommendations was the role of the geriatric service in screening, identifying, and managing the frail patient. Multidisciplinary teams should consist of surgeons from various subspecialties as well as representatives from medical specialties (e.g., geriatric medicine, geriatric psychiatry, wound care, palliative care, physical medicine, and rehabilitation) [71].

Management of frailty includes the coupling of effective prevention with directed therapeutic approaches [72]. In one study, 188 frail people living at home were randomized to undergo either physical therapy-based intervention or an educational program (control group) [73]. The study showed improved functional outcomes in the intervention group. In addition, inactivity and muscle weakness have been found to be significantly associated with frailty [74].

In another study, there was a strong relationship between daily sedentary time and development of physical frailty [75]. This highlights the importance of physical and occupational therapy as critical components of the multidisciplinary approach to the management and prevention of frailty. It also supports the inclusion of social interventions to ensure that elderly patients stay active by participating in various activities or community work.

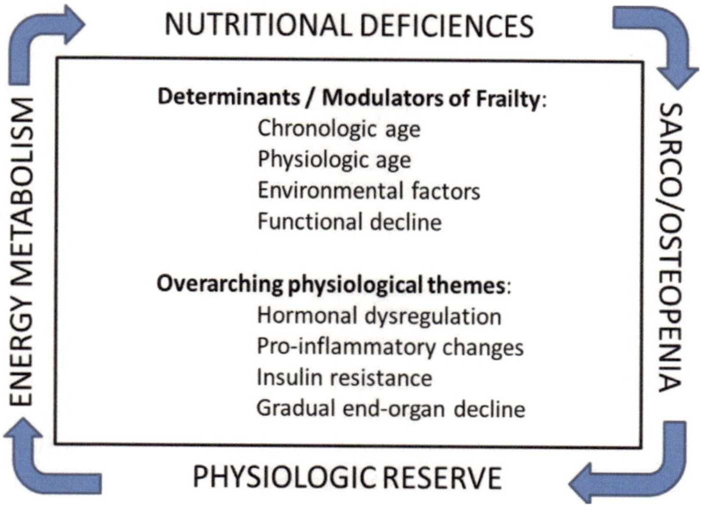

Figure 2. Major themes and manifestations associated with the development and progression of frailty. Modified with permission from McDermid et al. [124].

Major components of the frailty syndrome include weight loss [76], sarcopenia [77], and osteopenia [78, 79]. Consequently, adequate supplementation of protein, calories, and essential nutrients is important in the treatment and prevention of frailty [77]. At the same time, frailty can exist in the morbidly obese, corroborating the need for the multidisciplinary team approach [80]. In the context of osteopenia, it has been demonstrated that a simple intervention, such as vitamin D supplementation, has been shown to be beneficial in reducing hip fractures and associated complications in the frail, elderly patient [77, 81–84].

One randomized controlled trial evaluated the effects of nutritional, cognitive, physical, and combined interventions in frail, older adults. Combined approach utilizing physical exercise, nutritional supplementation, and cognitive training was effective in reducing frailty [85]. For some, advanced frailty is synonymous with the commonly used term, "failure to thrive". The main purpose of multi-pronged approaches is to prevent or delay the progression of frailty and to slow down the associated functional decline.

Polypharmacy has been proposed as an indirect reflection of frailty, especially when coupled with measures of comorbidity [33, 86, 58]. Significant correlations were found between CPS (Comorbidity-Polypharmacy Score) and a variety of clinical endpoints, including hospital readmissions, morbidity, mortality, and the need for discharge to skilled nursing facility [57–60]. Clinical data also suggest that CPS may indeed be a simplified surrogate of "frailty" [33,

58, 60]. The Beers criteria and STOPP and START criteria are tools to help reduce unnecessary pharmaceutical use in the frail population and may be helpful in preventing adverse medication events [87, 88]. In addition, the creation of geriatric units or treatment teams, with staff specifically trained to treat the frail and elderly, may help ensure that patients are not discharged from hospital on inappropriate medications.

Of importance, frail patients have been found to be more likely to use fall-risk-increasing drugs (FRIDs) as compared to their less frail counterparts, despite the danger of recurrent falls [89]. This further highlights the need to limit the use of unnecessary medications in the frail patient population. Although the responsibility for this rests primarily on the prescribing physician, visiting nurses and pharmacists could play an important role in monitoring for drug-drug interactions or inappropriate medication use. Given that there is a growing body of evidence to suggest that patients are more likely to be frail and suffer adverse outcomes if they have diseases such as cancer [90], renal failure [91], human immunodeficiency virus (HIV) [92], heart failure [93], or diabetes [94], it seems reasonable that the screening for, and identification of, frailty in these patient populations may lead to improved outcomes, more appropriate interventions, and better prevention.

In the emergency department (ED) setting, the challenge of screening for frailty is particularly difficult, given the time and resource constraints placed on emergency physicians and staff. One solution is the introduction of specialty teams of practitioners dedicated to assessing elderly patients arriving to the ED, resulting in the reduction of admissions from nursing homes [95]. Furthermore, if an elderly patient is evaluated by a geriatric team in the ED, they are more likely to be assessed using the CGA (Comprehensive Geriatric Assessment), and thus more readily identified, triaged, and cared for appropriately [96]. Specialty clinics dedicated to comprehensive and multidisciplinary assessment of frail older persons may be useful not only in terms of secondary prevention and management of frailty (and hence prevention of dependency) but also provide an opportunity for more aggressive monitoring and follow-up of this particular patient population as well as further research [97]. In summary, it is generally accepted that the identification and management of the frail patient should be overseen by dedicated specialty teams. Such teams should ideally consist of appropriately trained physicians, advanced practitioners, geriatric nurse specialists, physical therapists, pharmacists, and nutrition experts, and other health professionals.

6. Frailty: interventions and pitfalls

As we age, our bodies exhibit changes at both molecular and cellular levels. Some molecular changes are shared between tissue types and organ systems, whereas others are unique and specific. With advancing age, body composition changes, as evidenced by loss of muscle mass and increased percentage of body fat [98]. There is also a loss of bone mass, narrowing of joint spaces, and a decrease in total body water [98, 99]. Muscle mass may decrease by as much as 50% and body fat may increase to comprise up to 30% of body weight [99]. Once a "frail or pre-frail" individual is identified, it is critical to promptly begin interventions to slow down the progression of frailty. As outlined previously, these interventions should involve a well-coordinated, multidisciplinary approach. Key components of such a coordinated approach—physical activity, nutritional support, psycho-social support, and pharmaceutical management—are discussed.

Encouraging patients to remain active is among the most successful interventions to address frailty, both from the physical and cognitive perspective [100–102]. In a randomized study, 6 months of physical therapy reduced the functional decline of elderly patients living at home [74]. A meta-analysis investigating the impact of exercise on the quality of life in frail patients showed that exercise improves gait, balance, and performance of activities of daily living (ADLs) [103]. Of note, the majority of available research in this area involves supervised, short-term exercise regimens, making it difficult to generalize results to other settings. Furthermore, not all interventions were equally effective, with only three out of eight specific interventions reporting positive results in one analysis [104]. Finally, it is important for clinicians to determine if the patient is physically ready to begin exercise routines before proceeding, with emphasis being placed on ensuring safe environment for physical activity [105].

The importance of key factors behind nutritional supplementation (e.g., caloric, protein, and essential nutrient intake) has been studied extensively in relation to frailty. One study found that decreased caloric intake (e.g., <21 kcal/kg), low protein, and vitamin D and vitamin E intake were all associated with frailty [106]. While research on nutritional supplementation is still limited in the frail population, it is known that protein supplementation in elderly can be beneficial [107]. At the same time, a multicenter trial found that vitamin D supplementation did not improve rehabilitation outcome in frail individuals following injury [108]. There is some evidence that regular consumption of polyunsaturated fatty acids (PUFA) may be of benefit in modifying cognitive decline associated with aging [109]. The clinician should remember that isolated dietary interventions are not sufficient to combat frailty. With much more research needed in this area, there is thus far no definitive demonstration of benefit of nutritional interventions on measures of disability [104].

Pharmaceutical interventions in the frail population have revolved around the use of targeted therapies, coupled with polypharmacy reduction [107, 110, 111]. Of note, targeted programs to reduce polypharmacy result in fewer adverse events and better clinical outcomes [112–114]. In terms of specific interventions, anabolic agents have been shown to increase muscle mass but failed to improve strength or function in elderly patients [107]. Important research in the area of frailty involves erythropoietin and its potential neuroprotective and regenerative properties [100], angiotensin-converting enzyme (ACE) inhibitors [115], hormone therapies [116], and other pharmaceutical interventions to reverse sarcopenia [117] and cognitive decline [118, 119].

Given the above information in aggregate, it is reasonable to state that multi-pronged, coordinated programs encompassing physical activity, social support, nutritional supplementation, and pharmacologic interventions will be more effective than isolated efforts in each of the above areas [100–102, 107, 110, 111, 120].

7. Frailty: focus on prevention and care optimization

In the context of prevention and care optimization, it is critical to define and quantify the types of adverse events that are more prevalent within the "frail" and "pre-frail" populations. For example, frailty is associated with various adverse occurrences such as falls, disability, and death [121, 122]. Frail patients are more susceptible to skeletal fractures, healthcare associated infections, delirium, incontinence, malnutrition, dehydration, and skin breakdown [121, 123]. These factors all directly and indirectly contribute to morbidity, disability, and mortality. Injury and acute illness have a disproportionate impact on frail patients because of the impaired healing process, slower physical recovery, and longer hospital and intensive care stays when compared to non-frail patients [124, 125]. Frail patients also have higher rates of functional dependence, hospital readmission, and are less likely to go back to independent living after discharge [57, 126]. Because this negative feedback cycle is often difficult to halt once it has begun, it is critical that early prevention is implemented. Promoting healthy and positive behaviors (e.g., physical activity, reducing tobacco/alcohol use), and ensuring adequate community support helps reduce the risk of adverse events [127, 128]. Because acute exacerbations of chronic illness such as diabetes, heart failure, and pulmonary disease can quickly trigger complications in frail patients, regular provision of preventive care and structured medical follow-up are vitally important [129].

As outlined in previous sections of this chapter, adequate nutrition is important to both prevention and recovery from various health crises. Physiological changes due to aging and comorbid illness predispose the older population to malnutrition [130, 131]. With this in mind, both identification and prevention of nutritional deficiencies become critical in the multipronged approach to the frail patient [132, 133]. Finally, whereas in the past there existed a clear separation between acute care (i.e., inpatient hospitals, outpatient clinics) and long-term care (i.e., retirement homes, assisted living, home health), skilled nursing facilities have gradually begun to provide subacute care and rehabilitation services [134, 135]. Assisted living has played a major role in caring for frail patients, with many assisted living facilities offering services such as medication management, skilled nursing care, and extensive functional support [136]. Also important is the rapidly evolving concept of "chronic critical illness" associated with prolonged recovery from serious illness in the setting of pre-existing or newly acquired frailty [137]. A new "level of care" in the health care continuum arose as a response to "chronic critical illness" in the form of Long-Term Acute Care units [137].

The Older Americans Act (OAA) defines a multipurpose senior center as "…a community facility for the organization and provision of a broad spectrum of services, which shall include provision of health (including mental health), social, nutritional, and educational services and the provision of facilities for recreational activities for older individuals" [138]. In 2011, the National Council on Aging (NCoA) issued a reauthorization of the Older Americans Act which focused on multipurpose senior centers for positive aging, proposing that existing senior centers modernize to foster innovation, leadership, and capacity-building [139]. Many facilities were recognized as centers for positive aging even before the reauthorization. These centers feature specialty teams consisting of geriatricians, nurse practitioners, and social workers who provide consultations, comprehensive evaluations, and recommendations for senior care.

These teams work with patients, family members, and primary care providers to evaluate the patient's physical, emotional, social, and functional needs and assist in planning for the future [140].

Aging is associated with physical, psychological, and social factors that collectively contribute to the development of dependence. Consequently, frail patients should be encouraged to take active part in their own medical care. Active patient participation allows medical staff, caretakers, and family members to better understand expectations, goals of care, and treatment outcomes. The introduction of electronic health records allows patients to become engaged in their own care [141]. It is hoped that patient participation in self-management programs can translate into better outcomes, especially for the frail and elderly patients [142].

8. Rehabilitation: managing the frail patient

Injury and acute illness among older adults, frail or not, is always a significant event. Because functional capacity is likely to further decline following injury or acute illness, rehabilitation is of utmost importance in this setting, especially for older, frail patients [143]. To maximize rehabilitation potential, a multidisciplinary approach involving coordinated medical and nursing care appears to be the most effective way of optimizing the patient's functional status [144].

Because severe cognitive impairment is associated with poor functional recovery, individuals who fall into this category require special attention [145, 146]. Cognitive tests to determine baseline status and to predict potential for improvement may be helpful [147]. Of note, individuals with below average functional status at baseline have the most to gain from rehabilitation. In a society in which length and type of medical care are determined with cost in mind, caution must be taken to prevent short-term cost-saving measures from compromising long-term outcomes in frail patients undergoing rehabilitation [144, 148].

In order to create an environment where frail patients can thrive, it is important to focus on preventing adverse events (and other factors) that may negatively affect the recovery and rehabilitation process. Depression and cognitive impairment correlate with negative outcomes in elderly patients undergoing rehabilitation [149, 150]. In addition, pressure ulcers, urinary incontinence, and hearing impairment, when present, may further worsen the overall functional decline [151]. Many of these factors can be prevented, treated, or otherwise modified by leveraging various ancillary services to improve outcomes [152]. Patients who are unable to control their bowel and bladder function greatly benefit from interventions (i.e., rotation, pressure pads, etc.) that prevent pressure ulcers [153].

9. Miscellaneous topics: futility, delirium, and cognitive decline

The challenges with futility often have as much to do with the care provider as with the patient [154]. It is generally difficult to achieve agreement among providers caring for an individual and between different specialties consulting on the same patient. Further complicating these situations is the transition from "generally well" to "functional ill" to "not well/frail" to "acutely sick/dying" [155]. As physicians, we may be able to "see" the differences, but the family may simply see their very sick loved one still connected to "all of those machines/drips/monitors", yet not necessarily grasping the true severity of illness [156]. It is often difficult to achieve adequate understanding of futility after the intensive care team has been employing aggressive management approaches for days, weeks, or even months [157, 158].

Additional level of complexity emerges due to the lack of universal, legal definition of futility and state-to-state variations regarding existing options and responsibilities [159]. For example, Texas has a well-defined (but still controversial) futility statute [160, 161], while other localities have no formal statutes recognizing (or defining) futility [162]. Most biomedical ethicists support the autonomy of an individual physician to refuse a treatment or procedure that he or she is morally, ethically, or religiously opposed to (or feels that it would cause undue harm to the patient). In exchange, that physician has an obligation to refer the patient to another provider [163]. Abandonment, without transferring care to another competent individual, is never an option [164]. When approaching a futile situation, key questions need to be answered in order to better guide the course of goals-of-care discussions and subsequent magnitude of therapeutic interventions: (a) What are the values of the patient/family? (b) What gives meaning to a life of the patient and his/her family? (c) What qualities/aspects of care would represent unacceptable burdens? (d) What are the patient's hopes and fears?

Important considerations for individual providers include (a) clarity over what is determined to be futile; (b) the ability to recognize own biases, especially in the context of a futile situation; (c) maintenance of consistent communication within the team and with the patient/family; (d) having an accurate assessment of patient understanding and competence/capacity; (e) providing consistent palliation/palliative care (understanding physical, emotional, social, and spiritual aspects); and (f) consideration of all available options including hospice care when meeting with the patient and his/her family. A summary of the above considerations is provided in **Table 2**.

One should initiate the discussion about futility by providing an honest and realistic assessment of the medical situation [165]. A parallel assessment of the patient/family's values and goals of care is also made during the process. The ability to establish a collaborative working relationship between the health care team and the patient/family will help facilitate subsequent understanding in case that any future aggressive care becomes futile, and a strictly palliative approach (e.g., hospice) is more in keeping with patient/family goals [166, 167]. Of importance, key ethical principles of autonomy, beneficence, non-maleficence, and justice must be embedded throughout the entire process [168–170]. Together, these principles can help guide the creation of a rational plan of care [168–170]. Considering the unit of care as the "patient-family" as opposed to just the patient may also broaden our understanding of unique dynamics that may influence the decision-making process. Defining futility, especially in the geriatric population, must include a broad-based assessment consisting of the following key elements [154, 171–173]:

Communication considerations

Ask-Tell-Ask: Do not make any assumptions. Answer honestly and directly.

Sit-Listen-Make eye contact: Make sure that everyone is there who needs to be there.

SPIKES: Set up, Perception, Invitation, Knowledge, Emotions, Strategy/Summary.

Address emotion: Name; Understand; Respect; Support; Explore

Advance care planning: Start early; Review with any change in status/level of care; Know applicable status levels; Conversations now a billable visit under Medicare regulations.

Living will versus advance directive

Durable power of attorney for health

Guardianship—If no other acceptable options exist, consider sooner than later if patient lacks capacity or competence and no other documents have been completed.

POLST—Physician Orders for Life-Sustaining Treatment should be completed for anyone with frailty or anyone in whom you would not be surprised if they were to die within the next year.

Risk of abuse and social vulnerability

Frailty increases the risk of abuse

Prevention and education

Working closely with patients and families

Available programs and organizations

Compiled from Eng et al. (1997) *J Am Geriatr Soc* 45(2):223–232 ; Evans et al. (2006) *The Cancer Journal*12(5): 417–424; Harris (2007) *Postgraduate Obstetrics & Gynecology*27(4): 1–4; Wittenberg-Lyles et al. (2008) *Social Science & Medicine* 66(11): 2356–2365.

Table 2. Important considerations and concepts when communicating about frailty and related issues, including end-of-life issues.

- *Patient factors*: (a) comorbid medical conditions; (b) functional capacity (e.g., Karnofsky/Palliative Performance Scale or PPS [174]); (c) medication profile; (d) competence/mental capacity [175]; (d) quality of life; (e) overall goals and values; (f) documented wishes (advance directive/living will/Physician Orders for Life-Sustaining Treatment (POLST) [176])

- *Social and cultural factors*: (a) Where does the patient live? (b) Who does the patient live with? (c) Who helps them, including decisional support? (d) What are their financial resources or limitations? (e) What is the patient's access to care? Available transportation? (f) What is the patient's cultural/ethnic background? (g) Regarding community resources, who is in the "extended family"? (h) Is the patient safe? Is there any potential for abuse?

- *Emotional factors*: (a) Is there an underlying metal illness? (b) Is there an underlying substance abuse/addiction? (c) Is there a suspicion of elder abuse or neglect? (d) Is loneliness/isolation an issue?

- *Spiritual/religious factors* [177]: (a) Is faith important to the patient/family? (b) How does faith or belief impact decision-making? (c) Does the patient have a faith community?

Communication about futility should begin well before the "futility line" is crossed. It is important to consider the whole person when discussing subjects such as living wills and advance directives, and the conversation should be as much about the value, meaning, and quality of life as it is about whether to resuscitate someone [178]. Framing a conversation around realistic hopes and goals enables the patient and his/her family to clearly identify appropriate goals of care and, when appropriate, initiate discussions about palliative care, hospice, and Physician Orders for Life-Sustaining Treatment (POLST [179]) with a goal of avoiding unwanted medical situations (e.g., hospitalization, intensive care stays, long-term dependence on nursing care, etc.) [180, 181]. Discussing how to live, for a frail elderly individual with multiple medical conditions, should also include conversations about how to die [182]. Asking people who they are and what is most important to them allows the practitioner to frame recommendations for care in terms of the patient's goals, and not in terms of aggressive treatments that may be more burdensome than beneficial. Also, framing the conversation around positives helps preserve dignity in end-of-life care (e.g., "hospice care can allow you to be at home with your family and be comfortable" versus "there is nothing more we can do for you so we are calling hospice") [183].

Aging is a loss of homeostasis, or a breakdown in maintenance of specific molecular structures and pathways. It is the inevitable consequence of evolved anatomy and physiology of an organism [184]. Determining what constitutes normal aging and whether a decline in functional ability is attributable to disease or pathology can be challenging. While a series of changes occur with "normal" aging, a major characteristic of aging is the heterogeneity among the rates of functional decline [99].Time, genetics, disease, environmental, and behavioral factors all contribute to aging and frailty [185–188].The human body maintains significant reserve capacity, allowing individuals to endure and overcome a great deal of stress. Aging lowers the ceiling for an organ's or individual's reserve, and older adults have a lowered maximal capability when compared to younger individuals [99]. Thus, biologic age (represented by frailty), based on an individual's functional capacity, and not chronologic age, is the more optimal metric for studying the phenomenon of aging. Functional capacity is a direct measure of the ability of cells, tissues, and organ systems to function properly and optimally, and is influenced by both genes and environment[185–188]. Gradual changes in cells, tissues, and organs of the body lead to the eventual breakdown of maintenance processes—an inevitable consequence of the evolved anatomy and physiology of the organism [184].

10. Conclusions

As the geriatric segment of the world population continues to grow, the topic of frailty is bound to gain prominence around the globe. Despite significant amount of research available in this area, better understanding of frailty and its underlying mechanisms is required. The concept of frailty has evolved significantly since the mid-twentieth century, from the stereotypical description of a "thin, stooped, slow octogenarian" [7] to more contemporary definitions grounded in scientific evidence and practice. In this chapter, we reviewed some of the key issues that practitioners may encounter when treating frail patients, including identification of frailty, preventive and therapeutic options, common pitfalls, and related topics, including an overview of "goals of care"/end-of-life considerations.

Author details

Marissa S. Cohen[1], Elisabeth Paul[2], John David Nuschke[3], Julia C. Tolentino[4],
Ana V. Castellanos Mendez[5], Alaa-Eldin A. Mira[5], Ric A. Baxter[6] and Stanislaw P. Stawicki[7*]

*Address all correspondence to: stanislaw.stawicki@sluhn.org

1 Department of Emergency Medicine, St. Luke's University Health Network, Bethlehem, Pennsylvania, USA

2 Department of Internal Medicine, St. Luke's University Health Network, Bethlehem, Pennsylvania, USA

3 Temple University School of Medicine, St. Luke's University Hospital Campus, Bethlehem, Pennsylvania, USA

4 Department of Surgery, St. Luke's University Health Network, Bethlehem, Pennsylvania, USA

5 Department of Geriatric Medicine, St. Luke's University Health Network, Bethlehem, Pennsylvania, USA

6 Department of Palliative Medicine, St. Luke's University Health Network, Bethlehem, Pennsylvania, USA

7 Department of Research & Innovation, St. Luke's University Health Network, Bethlehem, Pennsylvania, USA

References

[1] Kinsella, K.G. and D.R. Phillips, Global aging: The challenge of success. Vol. 60. 2005, Population Reference Bureau, Washington, DC, USA.

[2] Bray, F. and B. Møller, Predicting the future burden of cancer. Nature Reviews Cancer, 2006. 6(1): pp. 63–74.

[3] Hubbard, R.E., et al., Inflammation and frailty measures in older people. Journal of Cellular and Molecular Medicine, 2009. 13(9b): pp. 3103–3109.

[4] Hubbard, R.E., M.S. O'Mahony, and K.W. Woodhouse, Characterising frailty in the clinical setting—a comparison of different approaches. Age and Ageing, 2009. 38(1): pp. 115–119.

[5] Hubbard, R. and D. Story, Patient frailty: the elephant in the operating room. Anaesthesia, 2014. 69(s1): pp. 26–34.

[6] Nyland, J. and J.D. Abbott, Functional fitness, life stress, and transitions across the life span, in Handbook of Stressful Transitions Across the Lifespan. 2010, New York: Springer. pp. 605–623.

[7] Sternberg, S.A., et al., The identification of frailty: a systematic literature review. Journal of the American Geriatrics Society, 2011. 59(11): pp. 2129–2138.

[8] Old and frail. Br Med J, 1968. 1(5594): pp. 723–724.

[9] Pawlson, L.G., Hospital length of stay of frail elderly patients: primary care by general internists versus geriatricians. Journal of the American Geriatrics Society, 1988. 36(3): pp. 202–208.

[10] Milte, R. and M. Crotty, Musculoskeletal health, frailty and functional decline. Best Practice & Research Clinical Rheumatology, 2014. 28(3): pp. 395–410.

[11] Brown, I., R. Renwick, and D. Raphael, Frailty: constructing a common meaning, definition, and conceptual framework. International Journal of Rehabilitation Research, 1995. 18(2): pp. 93–102.

[12] Fried, L.P., et al., Frailty in older adults evidence for a phenotype. The Journals of Gerontology Series A: Biological Sciences and Medical Sciences, 2001. 56(3): pp. M146–M157.

[13] Rockwood, K., et al., Prevalence, attributes, and outcomes of fitness and frailty in community-dwelling older adults: report from the Canadian study of health and aging. The Journals of Gerontology Series A: Biological Sciences and Medical Sciences, 2004. 59(12): pp. 1310–1317.

[14] Rockwood, K., What would make a definition of frailty successful? Age and Ageing, 2005. 34(5): pp. 432–434.

[15] Boers, M. and A.J.C. Jentoft, A new concept of health can improve the definition of frailty. Calcified Tissue International, 2015. 97(5): pp. 429–431.

[16] Huber, M., et al., How should we define health? BMJ, 2011. 343.

[17] Berrut, G., et al., Promoting access to innovation for frail old persons. The Journal of Nutrition, Health & Aging, 2013. 17(8): pp. 688–693.

[18] Xue, Q.-L., The frailty syndrome: definition and natural history. Clinics in Geriatric Medicine, 2011. 27(1): pp. 1–15.

[19] Fried, L.P., et al., Untangling the concepts of disability, frailty, and comorbidity: implications for improved targeting and care. The Journals of Gerontology Series A: Biological Sciences and Medical Sciences, 2004. 59(3): pp. M255–M263.

[20] Sheaff, R., et al., Impacts of case management for frail elderly people: a qualitative study. Journal of Health Services Research & Policy, 2009. 14(2): pp. 88–95.

[21] Bihan, B.L. and C. Martin, A comparative case study of care systems for frail elderly people: Germany, Spain, France, Italy, United Kingdom and Sweden. Social Policy & Administration, 2006. 40(1): pp. 26–46.

[22] Afilalo, J., Frailty in patients with cardiovascular disease: why, when, and how to measure. Current Cardiovascular Risk Reports, 2011. 5(5): pp. 467–472.

[23] Revenig, L.M., et al., Too frail for surgery? Initial results of a large multidisciplinary prospective study examining preoperative variables predictive of poor surgical outcomes. Journal of the American College of Surgeons, 2013. 217(4): pp. 665–670. e1.

[24] Buigues, C., et al., Frailty syndrome and pre-operative risk evaluation: a systematic review. Archives of Gerontology and Geriatrics, 2015. 61(3): pp. 309–321.

[25] Wieland, D. and V. Hirth, Comprehensive geriatric assessment. Cancer Control: Journal of the Moffitt Cancer Center, 2002. 10(6): pp. 454–462.

[26] Tucci, A., et al., A comprehensive geriatric assessment is more effective than clinical judgment to identify elderly diffuse large cell lymphoma patients who benefit from aggressive therapy. Cancer, 2009. 115(19): pp. 4547–4553.

[27] Handforth, C., et al., The prevalence and outcomes of frailty in older cancer patients: a systematic review. Annals of Oncology, 2015. 26(6): pp. 1091–1101.

[28] Baijal, P. and V. Periyakoil, Understanding frailty in cancer patients. The Cancer Journal, 2014. 20(5): pp. 358–366.

[29] Abdelhafiz, A.H., et al., Hypoglycemia in older people-a less well recognized risk factor for frailty. Aging and Disease, 2015. 6(2): p. 156.

[30] White, H.D., et al., Frailty is associated with worse outcomes in non-ST-segment elevation acute coronary syndromes: insights from the TaRgeted platelet Inhibition to cLarify the Optimal strateGy to medicallY manage Acute Coronary Syndromes (TRILOGY ACS) trial. European Heart Journal: Acute Cardiovascular Care, 2016. 5(3): pp. 231–242.

[31] Espinoza, S. and J.D. Walston, Frailty in older adults: insights and interventions. Cleveland Clinic Journal of Medicine, 2005. 72(12): p. 1105.

[32] Hankes, D.D., Self-care: assessing the aged client's need for independence. Journal of Gerontological Nursing, 1984. 10(5): pp. 26–31.

[33] Stawicki, S.P., et al., Comorbidity polypharmacy score and its clinical utility: A pragmatic practitioner's perspective. Journal of Emergencies, Trauma and Shock, 2015. 8(4): pp. 224–231.

[34] Harrison, J.K., et al., Managing frailty as a long-term condition. Age and Ageing, 2015. 44(5): pp. 732–735.

[35] Scuffham, P., S. Chaplin, and R. Legood, Incidence and costs of unintentional falls in older people in the United Kingdom. Journal of Epidemiology and Community Health, 2003. 57(9): pp. 740–744.

[36] Leslie, D.L., et al., One-year health care costs associated with delirium in the elderly population. Archives of Internal Medicine, 2008. 168(1): pp. 27–32.

[37] Comas-Herrera, A., et al., Cognitive impairment in older people: future demand for long-term care services and the associated costs. International Journal of Geriatric Psychiatry, 2007. 22(10): pp. 1037–1045.

[38] Ghignone, F., et al., The assessment and management of older cancer patients: a SIOG surgical task force survey on surgeons' attitudes. European Journal of Surgical Oncology (EJSO), 2016. 42(2): pp. 297–302.

[39] Lee, L., G. Heckman, and F.J. Molnar, Frailty Identifying elderly patients at high risk of poor outcomes. Canadian Family Physician, 2015. 61(3): pp. 227–231.

[40] Clegg, A., et al., Frailty in elderly people. Lancet, 2013. 381(9868): pp. 752–762.

[41] Junius-Walker, U., et al., Health and treatment priorities in patients with multimorbidity: report on a workshop from the European General Practice Network meeting 'Research on multimorbidity in general practice'. The European Journal of General Practice, 2010. 16(1): pp. 51–54.

[42] Welsh, T., A.L. Gordon, and J. Gladman, Comprehensive geriatric assessment–a guide for the non-specialist. International Journal of Clinical Practice, 2014. 68(3): pp. 290–293.

[43] Ellis, G., et al., Comprehensive geriatric assessment for older adults admitted to hospital: meta-analysis of randomised controlled trials. BMJ, 2011. 343: p. d6553.

[44] Rockwood, K., et al., A global clinical measure of fitness and frailty in elderly people. CMAJ, 2005. 173(5): pp. 489–95.

[45] Fried, L.P., et al., From bedside to bench: research agenda for frailty. Science of Aging Knowledge Environment, 2005. 2005(31): p. pe24.

[46] Sternberg, S.A., et al., The identification of frailty: a systematic literature review. Journal of the American Geriatrics Society, 2011. 59(11): pp. 2129–2138.

[47] Amici, A., et al., Self-administrated test based on the Marigliano-Cacciafesta Polypathological Scale (MCPS), as a screening tool for early identification of frailty in the elderly: a cohort study. Archives of Gerontology and Geriatrics, 2011. 52(1): pp. e60–e65.

[48] Clegg, A., L. Rogers, and J. Young, Diagnostic test accuracy of simple instruments for identifying frailty in community-dwelling older people: a systematic review. Age and Ageing, 2015. 44(1): pp. 148–152..

[49] Illsley, A. and A. Clegg, Assessment of frailty in the inpatient setting. British Journal of Hospital Medicine (London), 2016. 77(1): pp. 29–32.

[50] Song, X., A. Mitnitski, and K. Rockwood, Prevalence and 10-year outcomes of frailty in older adults in relation to deficit accumulation. Journal of the American Geriatrics Society, 2010. 58(4): pp. 681–7.

[51] Bergman, H., et al., Frailty: an emerging research and clinical paradigm – issues and controversies. Journals of Gerontology Series A: Biological Sciences and Medical Sciences, 2007. 62(7): pp. 731–737.

[52] Charlson, M.E., et al., The Charlson comorbidity index is adapted to predict costs of chronic disease in primary care patients. Journal of Clinical Epidemiology, 2008. 61(12): pp. 1234–1240.

[53] Nuttall, M., J. van der Meulen, and M. Emberton, Charlson scores based on ICD-10 administrative data were valid in assessing comorbidity in patients undergoing urological cancer surgery. Journal of Clinical Epidemiology, 2006. 59(3): pp. 265–273.

[54] Elixhauser, A., et al., Comorbidity measures for use with administrative data. Medical Care, 1998. 36(1): pp. 8–27.

[55] van Walraven, C., et al., A modification of the Elixhauser comorbidity measures into a point system for hospital death using administrative data. Medical Care, 2009. 47(6): pp. 626–633.

[56] Evans, D.C., et al., Comorbidity-polypharmacy scoring facilitates outcome prediction in older trauma patients. Journal of the American Geriatrics Society, 2012. 60(8): pp. 1465–1470.

[57] Justiniano, C.F., et al., Comorbidity-polypharmacy score predicts in-hospital complications and the need for discharge to extended care facility in older burn patients. Journal of Burn Care and Research, 2015. 36(1): pp. 193–196.

[58] Housley, B.C., et al., Comorbidity-polypharmacy score predicts readmission in older trauma patients. Journal of Surgery Research, 2015. 199(1): pp. 237–243.

[59] Justiniano, C.F., et al., Comorbidity-polypharmacy score: a novel adjunct in post-emergency department trauma triage. Journal of Surgery Research, 2013. 181(1): pp. 16–19.

[60] Mubang, R.N., et al., Comorbidity-polypharmacy score as predictor of outcomes in older trauma patients: a retrospective validation study. World Journal of Surgery, 2015. 39(8): pp. 2068–2075.

[61] Chang, S.S., et al., Association between inflammatory-related disease burden and frailty: results from the Women's Health and Aging Studies (WHAS) I and II. Archives of Gerontology and Geriatrics, 2012. 54(1): pp. 9–15.

[62] Hubbard, R., et al., Effect of smoking on the accumulation of deficits, frailty and survival in older adults: a secondary analysis from the Canadian Study of Health and Aging. JNHA-The Journal of Nutrition, Health and Aging, 2009. 13(5): pp. 468–472.

[63] Spinewine, A., et al., Effect of a collaborative approach on the quality of prescribing for geriatric inpatients: a randomized, controlled trial. Journal of the American Geriatrics Society, 2007. 55(5): pp. 658–665.

[64] Chen, A., et al., Best practices in coordinated care. 2000, Mathematica Policy Research, Princeton, NJ.

[65] Sloan, J.P., Protocols in primary care geriatrics. 2012, New York: Springer. Science & Business Media.

[66] Anderson, E., Abstracts from the center to advance palliative care national seminar palliative care at the forefront: Innovation and opportunity. November 7–9, 2013, Dallas, Texas. Journal of Palliative Medicine. March, 2014. 17(3): A1–A26.

[67] Wagner, E.H., The role of patient care teams in chronic disease management. British Medical Journal, 2000. 320(7234): p. 569.

[68] Fried, L.P., Darer, J., and Walston, J. Frailty, in Geriatric Medicine. 2003: New York: Springer. pp. 1067–1076.

[69] Leipzig, R.M., W.J. Hall, and L.P. Fried, Treating our societal scotoma: the case for investing in geriatrics, our nation's future, and our patients. Annals of Internal Medicine, 2012. 156(9): pp. 657–659.

[70] Burton, J.R. and D.H. Solomon, Geriatric medicine: a true primary care discipline. Journal of the American Geriatrics Society, 1993. 41(4): pp. 459–462.

[71] Zenilman, M.E., M.R. Katlic, and R.A. Rosenthal, Geriatric surgery—evolution of a clinical community. The American Journal of Surgery, 2015. 209(6): pp. 943–949.

[72] Zuliani, G., et al., Counteracting inflammation and insulin resistance with diet and exercise: a strategy for frailty prevention? European Geriatric Medicine, 2015. 6(3): pp. 220–231.

[73] Gill, T.M., et al., A program to prevent functional decline in physically frail, elderly persons who live at home. New England Journal of Medicine, 2002. 347(14): pp. 1068–1074.

[74] Lally, F. and P. Crome, Understanding frailty. Postgraduate Medical Journal, 2007. 83(975): pp. 16–20.

[75] Song, J., et al., Sedentary behavior as a risk factor for physical frailty independent of moderate activity: results from the Osteoarthritis Initiative. American Journal of Public Health, 2015. 105(7): pp. 1439–1445.

[76] Martone, A.M., et al., Anorexia of aging: a modifiable risk factor for frailty. Nutrients, 2013. 5(10): pp. 4126–4133.

[77] Morley, J.E., et al., Nutritional recommendations for the management of sarcopenia. Journal of the American Medical Directors Association, 2010. 11(6): pp. 391–396.

[78] Russo, C.R., M. Ricca, and L. Ferrucci, True osteoporosis and frailty-related osteopenia: two different clinical entities. Journal of the American Geriatrics Society, 2000. 48(12): pp. 1738–1739.

[79] Topinková, E., Aging, disability and frailty. Annals of Nutrition and Metabolism, 2008. 52(Suppl. 1): pp. 6–11.

[80] Baumgartner, R.N., et al., Sarcopenic obesity predicts instrumental activities of daily living disability in the elderly. Obesity Research, 2004. 12(12): pp. 1995–2004.

[81] Murad, M.H., et al., The effect of vitamin D on falls: a systematic review and meta-analysis. The Journal of Clinical Endocrinology & Metabolism, 2011. 96(10): pp. 2997–3006.

[82] Bischoff-Ferrari, H.A., et al., A pooled analysis of vitamin D dose requirements for fracture prevention. New England Journal of Medicine, 2012. 367(1): pp. 40–49.

[83] Rejnmark, L., et al., Vitamin D with calcium reduces mortality: patient level pooled analysis of 70,528 patients from eight major vitamin D trials. The Journal of Clinical Endocrinology & Metabolism, 2012. 97(8): pp. 2670–2681.

[84] Morley, J.E., et al., Sarcopenia with limited mobility: an international consensus. Journal of the American Medical Directors Association, 2011. 12(6): pp. 403–409.

[85] Ng, T.P., et al., Nutritional, physical, cognitive, and combination interventions and frailty reversal among older adults: a randomized controlled trial. The American Journal of Medicine, 2015. 128(11): pp. 1225–1236. e1.

[86] Gnjidic, D., et al., High-risk prescribing and incidence of frailty among older community-dwelling men. Clinical Pharmacology & Therapeutics, 2012. 91(3): pp. 521–528.

[87] Resnick, B. and J.T. Pacala, 2012 Beers criteria. Journal of the American Geriatrics Society, 2012. 60(4): pp. 612–613.

[88] Gallagher, P., et al., STOPP (Screening Tool of Older Person's Prescriptions) and START (Screening Tool to Alert doctors to Right Treatment). Consensus validation. International Journal of Clinical Pharmacology and Therapeutics, 2008. 46(2): pp. 72–83.

[89] Bennett, A., et al., Prevalence and impact of fall-risk-increasing drugs, polypharmacy, and drug–drug interactions in robust versus frail hospitalised falls patients: a prospective cohort study. Drugs & Aging, 2014. 31(3): pp. 225–232.

[90] Ruiz, M., et al., Management of elderly and frail elderly cancer patients: the importance of comprehensive geriatrics assessment and the need for guidelines. The American Journal of the Medical Sciences, 2013. 346(1): pp. 66–69.

[91] Wilhelm-Leen, E.R., et al., Frailty and chronic kidney disease: the third national health and nutrition evaluation survey. The American Journal of Medicine, 2009. 122(7): pp. 664–671. e2.

[92] Desquilbet, L., et al., HIV-1 infection is associated with an earlier occurrence of a phenotype related to frailty. The Journals of Gerontology Series A: Biological Sciences and Medical Sciences, 2007. 62(11): pp. 1279–1286.

[93] Afilalo, J., et al., Role of frailty in patients with cardiovascular disease. The American Journal of Cardiology, 2009. 103(11): pp. 1616–1621.

[94] Sinclair, A.J., Diabetes in old age–changing concepts in the secondary care arena. Journal of the Royal College of Physicians, 2000. 34(3): pp. 240–244.

[95] Ellis, G., T. Marshall, and C. Ritchie, Comprehensive geriatric assessment in the emergency department. Clinical Interventions in Aging, 2014. 9: p. 2033.

[96] Oo, M., et al., Assessing frailty in the acute medical admission of elderly patients. The Journal of the Royal College of Physicians of Edinburgh, 2012. 43(4): pp. 301–308.

[97] Tavassoli, N., et al., Description of 1,108 older patients referred by their physician to the "Geriatric Frailty Clinic (GFC) for Assessment of Frailty and Prevention of Disability" at the Gerontopole. The Journal of Nutrition, Health & Aging, 2014. 18(5): pp. 457–464.

[98] Shi, S., K. Mörike, and U. Klotz, The clinical implications of ageing for rational drug therapy. European Journal of Clinical Pharmacology, 2008. 64(2): pp. 183–199.

[99] King, M. and M.S. Lipsky, Clinical implications of aging. Disease-a-Month: DM, 2015. 61(11): pp. 467–474.

[100] Walston, J., et al., Research agenda for frailty in older adults: toward a better understanding of physiology and etiology: summary from the American Geriatrics Society/National Institute on Aging Research Conference on Frailty in Older Adults. Journal of American Geriatrics Society, 2006. 54(6): pp. 991–1001.

[101] Binder, E.F., et al., Effects of progressive resistance training on body composition in frail older adults: results of a randomized, controlled trial. The Journals of Gerontology Series A: Biological Sciences and Medical Sciences, 2005. 60(11): pp. 1425–1431.

[102] GREIWE, J.S., et al., Resistance exercise decreases skeletal muscle tumor necrosis factor α in frail elderly humans. The FASEB Journal, 2001. 15(2): pp. 475–482.

[103] Chou, C.H., C.L. Hwang, and Y.T. Wu, Effect of exercise on physical function, daily living activities, and quality of life in the frail older adults: a meta-analysis. Archives of Physical Medicine and Rehabilitation, 2012. 93(2): pp. 237–44.

[104] Daniels, R., et al., Interventions to prevent disability in frail community-dwelling elderly: a systematic review. BMC Health Services Research, 2008. 8: p. 278.

[105] Heath, J.M. and M.R. Stuart, Prescribing exercise for frail elders. The Journal of the American Board of Family Practice, 2002. 15(3): pp. 218–228.

[106] Bartali, B., et al., Low nutrient intake is an essential component of frailty in older persons. Journals of Gerontology Series A: Biological Sciences and Medical Sciences, 2006. 61(6): pp. 589–593.

[107] Lee, P.-H., Y.-S. Lee, and D.-C. Chan, Interventions targeting geriatric frailty: a systemic review. Journal of Clinical Gerontology and Geriatrics, 2012. 3(2): pp. 47–52.

[108] Latham, N.K., et al., A randomized, controlled trial of quadriceps resistance exercise and vitamin D in frail older people: the Frailty Interventions Trial in Elderly Subjects (FITNESS). Journal of the American Geriatrics Society, 2003. 51(3): pp. 291–299.

[109] Carrié, I., et al., PUFA for prevention and treatment of dementia? Current Pharmaceutical Design, 2009. 15(36): p. 4173.

[110] Morley, J.E., et al., Frailty consensus: a call to action. Journal of the American Medical Directors Association, 2013. 14(6): pp. 392–397.

[111] Birriel, T.J., et al., Adverse drug reactions in the era of multi-morbidity and polypharmacy. Journal of Basic and Clinical Pharmacy, 2015. 6(4): pp. 122–123.

[112] Milton, J.C. and S.H. Jackson, Inappropriate polypharmacy: reducing the burden of multiple medication. Clinical Medicine, 2007. 7(5): pp. 514–517.

[113] Hilmer, S.N., D. Gnjidic, and D.G. Le Couteur, Thinking through the medication list: appropriate prescribing and deprescribing in robust and frail older patients. Australian Family Physician, 2012. 41(12): p. 924.

[114] Hajjar, E.R., et al., Unnecessary drug use in frail older people at hospital discharge. Journal of the American Geriatrics Society, 2005. 53(9): pp. 1518–1523.

[115] Gray, S.L., et al., Angiotensin-converting enzyme inhibitor use and incident frailty in women aged 65 and older: prospective findings from the Women's Health Initiative Observational Study. Journal of the American Geriatrics Society, 2009. 57(2): pp. 297–303.

[116] Sambrook, P.N., et al., Serum parathyroid hormone is associated with increased mortality independent of 25-hydroxy vitamin d status, bone mass, and renal function in the frail and very old: a cohort study. Journal of Clinical Endocrinology and Metabolism, 2004. 89(11): pp. 5477–5481.

[117] Vellas, B., et al., Designing pharmaceutical trials for sarcopenia in frail older adults: EU/US Task Force recommendations. The Journal of Nutrition, Health & Aging, 2013. 17(7): pp. 612–618.

[118] Middleton, L.E. and K. Yaffe, Promising strategies for the prevention of dementia. Archives of Neurology, 2009. 66(10): pp. 1210–1215.

[119] Carrillo, M.C., et al., Can we prevent Alzheimer's disease? Secondary "prevention" trials in Alzheimer's disease. Alzheimer's & Dementia, 2013. 9(2): pp. 123–131. e1.

[120] Ekdahl, A.W., et al., Long-term evaluation of the ambulatory geriatric assessment: a frailty intervention trial (AGe-FIT): clinical outcomes and total costs after 36 months. Journal of the American Medical Directors Association, 2016. 17(3): pp. 263–8.

[121] Joosten, E., et al., Prevalence of frailty and its ability to predict in hospital delirium, falls, and 6-month mortality in hospitalized older patients. BMC Geriatrics, 2014. 14(1): p. 1.

[122] Spaniolas, K., et al., Ground level falls are associated with significant mortality in elderly patients. Journal of Trauma and Acute Care Surgery, 2010. 69(4): pp. 821–825.

[123] Laurila, J.V., et al., Predisposing and precipitating factors for delirium in a frail geriatric population. Journal of Psychosomatic Research, 2008. 65(3): pp. 249–254.

[124] McDermid, R.C., H.T. Stelfox, and S.M. Bagshaw, Frailty in the critically ill: a novel concept. Critical Care, 2011. 15(1): p. 301.

[125] Stawicki, S.P., et al., Rib fractures in the elderly: a marker of injury severity. Journal of the American Geriatrics Society, 2004. 52(5): pp. 805–808.

[126] Bagshaw, S.M., et al., Association between frailty and short-and long-term outcomes among critically ill patients: a multicentre prospective cohort study. Canadian Medical Association Journal, 2014. 186(2): pp. E95–E102.

[127] Oliver, D., C. Foot, and R. Humphries, Making our health and care systems fit for an ageing population. 2014, The King's Fund, London.

[128] Downs, M. and B. Bowers, Excellence in dementia care: research into practice. 2014, UK, McGraw-Hill Education.

[129] Purdy, S., et al., Interventions to reduce unplanned hospital admission. Bristol, United Kingdom: National Institute for Health Research, 2012. Available from http://www.bristol.ac.uk/media-library/sites/primaryhealthcare/migrated/documents/unplannedadmissions.pdf.

[130] Seiler, W.O., Clinical pictures of malnutrition in ill elderly subjects. Nutrition, 2001. 17(6): pp. 496–498.

[131] Landi, F., et al., Body mass index and mortality among older people living in the community. Journal of the American Geriatrics Society, 1999. 47(9): pp. 1072–1076.

[132] Wells, J.L. and A.C. Dumbrell, Nutrition and aging: assessment and treatment of compromised nutritional status in frail elderly patients. Clinical Interventions in Aging, 2006. 1(1): pp. 67–79.

[133] Bukata, S.V., et al., A guide to improving the care of patients with fragility fractures. Geriatric Orthopaedic Surgery and Rehabilitation, 2011. 2(1): pp. 5–37.

[134] Jette, D.U., R.L. Warren, and C. Wirtalla, The relation between therapy intensity and outcomes of rehabilitation in skilled nursing facilities. Archives of Physical Medicine and Rehabilitation, 2005. 86(3): pp. 373–379.

[135] Jette, D.U., R.L. Warren, and C. Wirtalla, Rehabilitation in skilled nursing facilities: effect of nursing staff level and therapy intensity on outcomes. American Journal of Physical Medicine & Rehabilitation, 2004. 83(9): pp. 704–712.

[136] Gelhaus, L., More reasons to stay. Increasing services such as medication management and extra assistance with ADLs leads assisted living providers into uncharted territory. Provider, 2001. 27(8): pp. 18–20, 23, 26–8.

[137] Baldwin M.R., Reid M.C., Westlake A.A., Rowe J.W., Granieri E.C., Wunsch H., Dam T.T., Rabinowitz D., Goldstein N.E., Maurer M.S., Lederer D.J. The feasibility of measuring frailty to predict disability and mortality in older medical intensive care unit survivors. Journal of Critical Care. 2014 Jun 30;29(3):401–8.

[138] Turner, K.W., Senior citizens centers: What they offer, who participates, and what they gain. Journal of Gerontological Social Work, 2004. 43(1): pp. 37–47.

[139] National Council on Aging. [2015 April 1, 2016]; Available from: https://www.ncoa.org/.

[140] St. Luke's University Health Network. St. Luke's Opens Center for Positive Aging in Bethlehem. [2015 April 1, 2016]; Available from: http://www.slhn.org/News/2014/Center-for-Positive-Aging-Opens-in-Bethlehem.

[141] Hatcher, M., Intranet usage and potential in acute care hospitals in the United States: survey-2000. Journal of Medical Systems, 2001. 25(6): pp. 345–355.

[142] Lorig, K.R., et al., Evidence suggesting that a chronic disease self-management program can improve health status while reducing hospitalization: a randomized trial. Medical Care, 1999. 37(1): pp. 5–14.

[143] Kelley-Quon, L., et al., Functional status after injury: a longitudinal study of geriatric trauma. The American Surgeon, 2010. 76(10): p. 1055.

[144] Lyons, A.R., Clinical outcomes and treatment of hip fractures. The American Journal of Medicine, 1997. 103(2A): pp. 51S–63S; discussion 63S–64S.

[145] Landi, F., et al., Predictors of rehabilitation outcomes in frail patients treated in a geriatric hospital. Journal of the American Geriatrics Society, 2002. 50(4): pp. 679–684.

[146] Tripathi, R.S., et al., An iatrogenic metabolic encephalopathy in a nonagenarian: the dilemma of a critical miss as a possible social dismissal. International Journal of Critical Illness and Injury Science, 2013. 3(4): p. 282.

[147] Heruti, R.J., et al., Rehabilitation outcome of elderly patients after a first stroke: effect of cognitive status at admission on the functional outcome. Archives of Physical Medicine and Rehabilitation, 2002. 83(6): pp. 742–749.

[148] Papadimos, T.J. and S.P. Stawicki, The aging paradox: how old is old and all that jazz? Journal of the American Geriatrics Society, 2011. 59(10): pp. 1987–1988.

[149] Lenze, E.J., et al., Adverse effects of depression and cognitive impairment on rehabilitation participation and recovery from hip fracture. International Journal of Geriatric Psychiatry, 2004. 19(5): pp. 472–478.

[150] Fusco, D., et al., Predictors of rehabilitation outcome among frail elderly patients living in the community. Journal of the American Medical Directors Association, 2009. 10(5): pp. 335–341.

[151] Landi, F., et al., Functional decline in frail community-dwelling stroke patients. European Journal of Neurology, 2006. 13(1): pp. 17–23.

[152] Bernabei, R., et al., The comprehensive geriatric assessment: when, where, how. Critical Reviews in Oncology/Hematology, 2000. 33(1): pp. 45–56.

[153] Reilly, E.F., et al., Pressure ulcers in the intensive care unit: The 'forgotten'enemy. OPUS 12 Scientist, 2007. 1(2): pp. 17–30.

[154] Schneiderman, L.J., N.S. Jecker, and A.R. Jonsen, Medical futility: its meaning and ethical implications. Annals of Internal Medicine, 1990. 112(12): pp. 949–954.

[155] Gubrium, J.F. and J.A. Holstein, The nursing home as a discursive anchor for the ageing body. Ageing and Society, 1999. 19(5): pp. 519–538.

[156] Lee, D.K., et al., Withdrawing care: experience in a medical intensive care unit. JAMA, 1994. 271(17): pp. 1358–1361.

[157] Mizrahi, T. and J.S. Abramson, Sources of strain between physicians and social workers: implications for social workers in health care settings. Social Work in Health Care, 1985. 10(3): pp. 33–51.

[158] Solomon, M.Z., How physicians talk about futility: making words mean too many things. The Journal of Law, Medicine & Ethics, 1993. 21(2): pp. 231–237.

[159] Rowland, B., Communicating past and conflict: solving the medical futility controversy with process-based approached. University of Miami International and Comparative Law Review, 2006. 14: p. 271.

[160] Fine, R.L. and T.W. Mayo, Resolution of futility by due process: early experience with the Texas Advance Directives Act. Annals of Internal Medicine, 2003. 138(9): pp. 743–746.

[161] Truog, R.D., Counterpoint: the Texas advance directives act is ethically flawed: medical futility disputes must be resolved by a fair process. CHEST Journal, 2009. 136(4): pp. 968–971.

[162] Pope, T.M., Medical futility statutes: no safe harbor to unilaterally refuse life-sustaining treatment. Tennessee Law Review, 2007. 75(1): pp. 1–81.

[163] Luce, J.M., Physicians do not have a responsibility to provide futile or unreasonable care if a patient or family insists. Critical Care Medicine, 1995. 23(4): pp. 760–766.

[164] Pellegrino, E.D., Patient and physician autonomy: conflicting rights and obligations in the physician-patient relationship. The Journal of Contemporary Health Law and Policy, 1994. 10: p. 47.

[165] Papadimos, T.J., et al., Diagnosing dying. Anesthesia & Analgesia, 2014. 118(4): pp. 879–882.

[166] Towle, A. and W. Godolphin, Framework for teaching and learning informed shared decision making. British Medical Journal, 1999. 319(7212): p. 766.

[167] Ford, P.J., et al., Anti-infective therapy at end of life: Ethical decision-making in hospice-eligible patients. Bioethics, 2005. 19(4): pp. 379–392.

[168] Winter, B. and S. Cohen, ABC of intensive care: withdrawal of treatment. British Medical Journal, 1999. 319(7205): p. 306.

[169] Kinlaw, K. Ethical issues in palliative care. Semin Oncol Nurs, 2005. 21(1): pp. 63–68.

[170] Pellegrino, E.D. and D.C. Thomasma, Conflict between autonomy and beneficence in medical ethics: proposal for a resolution, The Journal of Contemporary Health Law and Policy, 1987. 3: p. 23.

[171] Post, S.G., C.M. Puchalski, and D.B. Larson, Physicians and patient spirituality: professional boundaries, competency, and ethics. Annals of Internal Medicine, 2000. 132(7): pp. 578–583.

[172] Frick, S., D.E. Uehlinger, and R.M.Z. Zenklusen, Medical futility: Predicting outcome of intensive care unit patients by nurses and doctors—a prospective comparative study. Critical Care Medicine, 2003. 31(2): pp. 456–461.

[173] Miettinen, T.T. and R.S. Tilvis, Medical futility as a cause of suffering of dying patients – the family members' perspective. Journal of Palliative Care, 1999. 15(2): p. 26.

[174] Kring, D.L. and P. Crane, Predictors of the end of life in chronic kidney disease: A pilot study. Southern Online Journal of Nursing Research, 2007. 9(3): pp. 1–8.

[175] Appelbaum, P.S. and T. Grisso, Assessing patients' capacities to consent to treatment. New England Journal of Medicine, 1988. 319(25): pp. 1635–1638.

[176] Hickman, S.E., et al., Hope for the future: achieving the original intent of advance directives. The Hastings Center Report, 2005: pp. S26–S30.

[177] Cavalieri, T.A., Ethical issues at the end of life. The Journal of the American Osteopathic Association, 2001. 101(10): pp. 616–624.

[178] Doukas, D.J. and L.B. McCullough, The values history: The evaluation of the patient's values and advance directives. Journal of Family Practice, 1991. 32(2): pp. 145–154.

[179] Hickman, S.E., et al., The POLST (Physician Orders for Life-Sustaining Treatment) paradigm to improve end-of-life care: potential state legal barriers to implementation. The Journal of Law, Medicine & Ethics, 2008. 36(1): pp. 119–140.

[180] Lawton, J., The dying process: patients' experiences of palliative care. 2002, New York: Routledge.

[181] Oliver, D.P., D. Porock, and S. Zweig, End-of-life care in US nursing homes: a review of the evidence. Journal of the American Medical Directors Association, 2005. 6(3): pp. S21–S30.

[182] Hanson, L.C., M. Danis, and J. Garrett, What is wrong with end-of-life care? Opinions of bereaved family members. Journal of the American Geriatrics Society, 1997. 45(11): pp. 1339–1344.

[183] Brown, H., B. Johnston, and U. Östlund, Identifying care actions to conserve dignity in end-of-life care. British Journal of Community Nursing, 2011. 16(5): pp. 238–245.

[184] Geriatrics review syllabus: a core curriculum in geriatric medicine. 8th ed. 2013, American Geriatrics Society, New York, NY

[185] Mattson, M.P., S.L. Chan, and W. Duan, Modification of brain aging and neurodegenerative disorders by genes, diet, and behavior. Physiological Reviews, 2002. 82(3): pp. 637–672.

[186] Boomsma, D., A. Busjahn, and L. Peltonen, Classical twin studies and beyond. Nature Reviews Genetics, 2002. 3(11): pp. 872–882.

[187] Williams, M.E., Clinical implications of aging physiology. The American Journal of Medicine, 1984. 76(6): pp. 1049–1054.

[188] Harris, T.B., et al., Age, gene/environment susceptibility–Reykjavik Study: multidisciplinary applied phenomics. American Journal of Epidemiology, 2007. 165(9): pp. 1076–1087.

Chapter 3

Assessment and Management of Older People in the General Hospital Setting

Inderpal Singh

Additional information is available at the end of the chapter

http://dx.doi.org/10.5772/64294

Abstract

Worldwide, populations are ageing. Older people, particularly centurions, represent the fastest growing sector and are counted as the success of the society. But not everyone ages successfully and enjoys good health. Many older people have multiple long-term medical, physical, mental, psychological and social problems. This can result in reduced quality of life, higher cost and poorer health outcome including increased mortality. Chronic diseases are associated with disability and low self-reported general health. In addition, physiological changes of ageing and consequent loss of functional reserve of the organ systems lead to the increased physical disability and dependency. Therefore, geriatric medicine could warrant a more holistic approach than general adult medicine. Nearly two-thirds of people admitted to hospital are over 65 years old and an increasing number are frail or have a diagnosis of dementia [1]. Our current training not only generates relatively low number of geriatricians but there also remains a huge need for better staff training and support to provide safe, holistic and dignified care. The cornerstone of modern geriatric medicine is the comprehensive geriatric assessment (CGA). This is defined as multidimensional, interdisciplinary diagnostic process that aims to determine a frail older person's medical conditions, mental health, functional capability and social circumstances in order to develop a coordinated and integrated plan for treatment, rehabilitation and long-term follow-up [2]. All older people admitted to hospital with an acute medical illness, geriatric syndromes including falls, incontinence, delirium or immobility, unexplained functional dependency or need for rehabilitation warrant CGA. CGA could screen for treatable illnesses, establish the key diagnosis leading to hospital admission and formulate a rational therapeutic plan thus resulting in the improved outcome. This chapter starts with an introduction to the ageing nation and impact of ageing on hospitals. This will be followed by discussing physiological changes of ageing and the various components of multidisciplinary assessment for older people admitted to hospital with an acute illness that could lead to high-level holistic care. It also covers a wide range of issues and challenges which medical team/multidisciplinary teams often come across during routine care of acutely unwell older people. The chapter concludes by a literature review on current evidence on the effectiveness of CGA and recommendations to enhance clinical care.

Keywords: Multidisciplinary, Secondary care, Polypharmacy, Nutrition, Co-morbidity

1. Introduction

Older people attending the emergency department (ED) or acute medical units (AMU) often have more complex needs due to multiple co-morbidities, physical limitations, increased functional dependence and complex psychosocial issues. Thus, they are more vulnerable and could easily decompensate with minor stressors, resulting in increased frailty. There are established detrimental effects of hospitalisation on older adults and about 17% of older medical patients who were independently mobile 2 weeks prior to hospital admission required assistance to walk at hospital discharge [3, 4]. Therefore, to improve outcomes for frail older people with multiple co-morbidities and an acute illness, admission should be to an Emergency Frailty Unit (EFU), a separate unit within an AMU but led by a geriatrician and the multidisciplinary team (MDT) to provide comprehensive person-centred care.

The clinical assessment of frail older people is challenging, as they often have multiple co-morbidities and diminished functional and physiological reserves. In addition, the physical illness or adverse effects of drugs are more pronounced resulting in atypical presentation, cognitive decline, delirium or inability to manage routine activities of daily living (ADLs) [5]. Among the potential adverse outcomes for frail older inpatients, are the risks of continued deterioration as a consequence of medical complications such as pressure sores, hospital-acquired infections or functional decline. This can also lead to long-term increased dependency, institutionalisation and death.

1.1. Impact of ageing on hospitals

Hospitals face a rising demand from an increasing number of acute emergency admissions of people aged 65 years and above with multiple co-morbidities and psychosocial problems. The admission rates for people over 65 years are three times higher than for people aged 16–64 years. Older patients cannot always be transferred quickly from the hospital after acute illness and on average hospital length of stay (LoS) is significantly higher than for under 65 years [6]. The older people occupy around two-thirds of acute hospital beds and emergency admissions have been rising for several years [7]. The healthcare cost and the proportion of hospital bed days used by older people are likely to increase further due to ageing population [8].

1.2. Physiological changes of ageing

The normal physiological changes occur with ageing in all organ systems (**Table 1**) and this has implications for the clinical assessment of older people [9–11]. Therefore, it is essential to be aware of these changes as these have an impact on drug metabolism and pharmacodynam-

http://dx.doi.org/10.5772/64294

ics. In addition to comprehensive geriatric assessment (CGA), these changes can be delayed or reversed with appropriate diet, exercise and medical intervention.

	Change in physiology	Impact on health
Cardiovascular	↓ Heart rate and cardiac output	Easy fatigability and loss of stamina for physical work
	↓ Arterial compliance	Peripheral oedema
	↑ Systolic blood pressure	Isolated systolic hypertension
	↑ Myocardial irritability	Dysrhythmias
	↓ Tissue perfusion	Cold sensitivity in the hands/feet
	↑ Circulation time	
Nervous system	↓ Normal reflexes	Impaired cognition
	↓ Proprioception	Falls
	↓ Baroreceptor response	Postural hypotension
	↓ Sympathetic response	
	↑ Sensitivity to anticholinergics	
Sensory	↓ Salivation and taste	Aspiration
	↓ Thirst	Dehydration
	↓ Response to pain	Falls
	↓ Visual acuity and peripheral vision	Increased isolation and depression
	↓ Hearing	
Lungs	↓ Tidal volume	Low oxygen saturations
	↓ Vital and total lung capacity	
	↓ Lung compliance	
	↓ Response to hypoxemia	
	↑ Residual volume	
Kidneys	↓ Glomerular filtration rate	Higher chance of drug side effects due to reduced renal clearance (serum creatinine level remains relatively constant due to reduced muscle mass and reduced creatinine production)
	↓ Renal flow and kidney size	
Bladder	Smaller voided volume	Urinary incontinence
	↓Bladder capacity	Urgency

	Change in physiology	Impact on health
	↑ Involuntary detrusor contractions	Overactive bladder symptoms
	↑ Residual volume	
Gastrointestinal	↓ Gastric emptying	Weight loss
	↓ Bowel movements	Constipation
	↓ Transit time and absorption	Slower drug metabolism and reduced hepatic first-pass effect, thus increased bioavailability
	↓ Liver mass (by 30-40%)	Dehydration
	↓ Sense of thirst	
	↓ Capacity to conserve water.	
Endocrine	↓ Insulin sensitivity	Hyperglycaemia during acute illness
	Thyroid impairment	Risk of hypothermia
	↓ Metabolic rate	Osteopenia/fragility fractures
	↓ Temperature regulation	
	↓ Bone mineral density	
Body composition	Atrophy of skin epidermis	Easy bruising
	↓ Subcutaneous fat	Pressure ulcers
	↓ Sweat glands	Dry skin
	Atrophy of muscle cells	Sarcopenia
	Degenerative changes in many joints	Falls
Immune system	↓ Neurohumoral response	Higher infection rate
	↓ T-cell response	Higher probability of infection

Table 1. Normal physiological changes of ageing.

2. Assessments of older people in hospital

The holistic assessment of older people is best achieved by the MDT. The MDT members include doctors, nurses, physiotherapist (PT), occupational therapist (OT), dietician, clinical pharmacist, social worker (SW), specialist nurses (e.g. tissue viability nurse and Parkinson's disease nurse specialist), hospital discharge liaison team and carers. Input from a clinical psychologist or old age psychiatrist may be needed depending on individual patients' needs. All members engage with patients and carers to complete their assessments and intervention, followed by multidisciplinary meeting (MDM) to formulate ongoing care plan and follow-up.

2.1. Medical assessment

The medical assessment begins at the time of admission to an AMU or an EFU with the appropriate investigations and thus establishing the relevant diagnosis. In addition to treating acute illness, there must be an attempt to optimise the symptoms and treatment of chronic diseases [12]. The common medical diseases among older people are listed in **Table 2**. A carer or a relative usually accompanies an older patient to the hospital, and a short conversation with them can rapidly reveal the diagnosis and direct ongoing management.

Mostly seen in older people	Alzheimer's disease
	Normal pressure hydrocephalus
	Temporal arteritis (giant cell arteritis)
	Diastolic heart failure
	Inclusion body myositis
	Atrophic urethritis and vaginitis
	Shingles (herpes zoster)
	Benign prostatic hyperplasia
	Aortic aneurysm
	Polymyalgia rheumatica
Common in older age group	Degenerative osteoarthritis
	Overactive bladder with urinary incontinence
	Diabetic hyperosmolar nonketotic coma
	Falls and fragility hip fracture
	Osteoporosis
	Parkinsonism
	Accidental hypothermia
	Pressure ulcers
	Prostate cancer
	Stroke
	Glaucoma and cataract
	Monoclonal gammopathies

Table 2. Common medical diseases among older people.

2.1.1. Acute medical illness

Older people admitted to the hospital with an acute illness often a non-specific presentation, which can obscure the serious underlying pathology or medical diagnosis. For example, acute bowel infarction in older people may not present with typical abdominal pain or tenderness or lack of typical signs on meningism in bacterial meningitis. The atypical presentation in older people could be one or combination of 'feeling unwell', 'inability to cope', 'off-legs', 'fall', 'confusion', 'dizziness', 'incontinence', 'weight loss', etc. The atypical presentation with possible background sensory impairment, lack of collateral history, polypharmacy and high prevalence of cognitive deficits limits good clinical assessment.

'Feeling unwell' or 'inability to cope' could be a presentation of an acute infection, exacerbation of underlying chronic disease (e.g. chronic heart failure), drug side effect (e.g. constipation) or dehydration. However, this could be due to underlying malignancy; therefore, such a presentation warrants good clinical examination and appropriate investigations.

Worldwide, falls are the second most common cause of unintentional injury and death. A non-accidental fall is a complex system failure in the human organ system, where a person comes to rest on the ground from a standing or a sitting height, unintentionally with no associated loss of consciousness [13]. The prevalence of falls increases with age, and oldest old is at highest risk. One-third of older adults over 65 years and half of older people above 80 years could experience one fall in a year [14, 15].

Falls are most common in institutionalised older people [16] and half of the fallers will fall again within a year [17]. Older people with high risk of falls are sometimes admitted to the hospital to avoid future falls but in reality, hospitals are associated with a higher risk of falling due to several new risk factors such as unfamiliar environment, increased risk of delirium, high beds, single rooms and so on [18, 19]. Falls are associated with a threefold increased risk of future falls, fear of falling, prolonged hospital stay, functional decline, increased dependency, institutionalisation, increased expenditure, morbidity and mortality [20, 21]. Falls result in injury (4%) and fragility hip fracture (1%), following which up to 10% of people will die within a month, a third dying during the following year after [22].

The evaluation of falls begins by distinguishing it from brief sudden loss of consciousness (syncope). However, it could be challenging to do so in certain cases but every effort should be made. Falls cannot only be simply related to underlying medical or neurological disorder as falls are usually multifactorial including a wide range of intrinsic and extrinsic factors. The most common factors leading to falls in neurological patients are the disorder of gait and balance (55%), epileptic seizures (12%), syncope (10%), stroke (7%) and dementia. Falls have particularly being linked to Parkinson's disease (62%), polyneuropathy (48%), epilepsy (41%), spinal disorders (41%), motor neuron disease (33%), multiple sclerosis (31%), psychogenic disorders (29%), stroke (22%) and patients with a pain syndrome (21%) [16]. Dementia is associated with impaired mobility and is an independent risk factor for falling [23]. People who present with a fall or report recurrent falls in the past year or demonstrate abnormalities of gait and/or balance should have multifactorial, multidisciplinary assessment for falls, risk factors, perceived functional abilities and fear of falling. In addition, bone health and history of previous fragility fractures should be explored [24].

'Delirium' is a common syndrome affecting older people admitted to AMU or EFU. It is a serious acute problem which has been best understood as an 'acute brain dysfunction' or an 'acute confusional state' characterised by a rapid onset of symptoms, fluctuating course and an altered level of consciousness, global disturbance of cognition or perceptual abnormalities.

The Diagnostic and Statistical Manual of Mental Disorders (DSM-IV-TR) defines delirium as 'a disturbance of consciousness that is accompanied by a change in cognition that cannot be better accounted for by a pre-existing or evolving dementia' [25].

The diagnosis of delirium is based on clinical observations, cognitive assessment, physical and neurological examination. Despite the common problem, delirium remains a major challenge and often under-diagnosed and poorly managed. Clinically, delirium can be divided into hyperactive, hypoactive or mixed forms, based on psychomotor behaviour. The Confusion Assessment Method (CAM) supports a diagnosis of delirium if there is a history of acute onset of confusion with a fluctuating course and inattention in the presence of either disorganised thinking and/or altered level of consciousness [26]. Collateral history from the family member or carers is helpful to detect a recent change in cognition.

Delirium usually occurs as a result of complex interactions among multiple risk factors such as cognitive impairment, Parkinson's disease, stroke, poor mobility, history of previous delirium, hearing or visual impairment, malnutrition or depression. It is often precipitated in the hospital setting due to acute medical illnesses including infection, acute coronary syndrome, bowel ischaemia, surgical disorder, polypharmacy, pain, dehydration, electrolyte imbalance, new environment, sleep deprivation, constipation, hypoxia, use of restraints or indwelling catheters.

Delirium, if not recognised early and managed appropriately, can result in poor outcomes, including prolonged hospital stay, increased functional dependence, institutionalisation, a risk of developing dementia, increased inpatient and post-discharge mortality [27–29]. Therefore, an older person admitted to hospital with confusion should be promptly assessed for delirium to improve clinical outcomes. The optimal assessment should be completed to identify underlying modifiable risk factors and treating precipitating factors, followed by reorientation and restoration of cognitive functions using non-pharmacological strategies including carer support and education, good communication among MDT and appropriate follow-up. The pharmacological drugs including haloperidol or risperidone should be used to manage severe agitation or behavioural disturbance.

'Dementia' is often recognised for the first time as an incidental condition when people are admitted to an acute hospital for another reason. More than one-third of acute medical admissions (42.4%) for over 70s have been reported to have dementia and only half of which were diagnosed prior to admission [30]. However, dementia can be misdiagnosed as an acute illness and can be accompanied by reversible cognitive decline. In addition, older people with known dementia who present with an altered mental state can be mislabelled as having progressed to another stage of dementia missing undiagnosed delirium. Older people with cognitive impairment are at increased risk of falls [31] and are also more likely to die during hospitalisation, and increased severity of cognitive impairment is associated with higher odds of mortality (from 2.7 in those with moderate impairment to 4.2 in those with severe impairment) [32]. Therefore, older people in hospital settings should be carefully assessed for underlying cognition. Dementia is a chronic progressive brain disorder marked by a disturbance of more than two domains of brain functions for more than 6 months. The various cognitive deficits may include short-term memory loss, language- or word-finding difficulties, mood and personality changes, impaired reasoning, learning new skills, inability to concentrate, plan or solve problems, difficulty in taking decisions or completing a task, disorientation, visuospatial difficulties or problems with calculations. Dementia is the most appropriate diagnosis when two or more cognitive deficits have an impact on ADLs or social interaction, often associated with behavioural and psychological symptoms of dementia (BPSD) [33].

'Frailty' is defined variably and there is no single generally accepted definition. Fried et al. [34] reported a clinical definition of frailty based on the presence of three or more frailty indicators: unintentional weight loss, slow walking speed, subjective exhaustion, low grip strength and low levels of physical activity. Frailty, based on these criteria, was predictive of poor outcome including institutionalisation and death [34]. Whereas Rockwood and Mitnitski [35] had advocated an alternative approach to frailty by considering frailty in relation to the accumulation of deficits with age, including medical, physical, functional, cognitive and nutritional problems. The frailty index expresses the number of deficits identified in an individual as a proportion of the total number of deficits considered. Higher values indicated a greater number of problems and hence greater frailty. For example, if 40 potential deficits were considered, and 10 were present in a given person, their frailty index would be 10/40 = 0.25 [36]. A valid index can be derived from the routine information collected on CGA [37–39]. Therefore, the presence of frailty on clinical judgement should prompt consideration to holistic assessment by MDT.

2.1.2. Chronic co-morbidities

Older people usually have more than five medical conditions and one pathological disorder in an organ, which can weaken another system. This results in increased disability, physical dependence, functional deterioration, isolation or even death. Long-term conditions in older people require very careful assessment and monitoring particularly whilst undergoing acute medical treatment in the hospital. Every older person admitted to MAU or EFU should have assessment of underlying chronic medical conditions, including ischaemic heart disease, heart failure, chronic respiratory diseases, chronic inflammatory and autoimmune problems. Modifiable cardiovascular risk factors such as diabetes mellitus, hypercholesterolemia, hypertension, obesity, excessive smoking or alcohol consumption should be reviewed and optimally addressed.

2.2. Mental health assessment

Many people with long-term physical health conditions also have mental health problems [40]. Mental health problems are common in older people, and 8–32% of patients admitted to acute hospitals were found to be depressed [41, 42]. Depression is not a natural part of ageing but can be easily missed in older patients, thus resulting in adverse outcome including delayed recovery and suicide. It is often reversible with early recognition and prompt intervention. Delirium has been reported in 27% of older patients above 70 years [41]. The prevalence of dementia in acute hospitals was reported as 48% in men and 75% in women older than 90 years [30].

The current service models for the provision of mental health input in general medical care wards are variable. The prevailing view in the United Kingdom is that old age psychiatrists have the main responsibility for the diagnosis and management of dementia and other mental health problems. In many hospitals, both psychiatric and medical notes are not easily accessible and are mostly kept separately [43].

The National Service Framework (UK) for older people was published in 2001—standard seven aims to promote good mental health in older people and to treat and support those older people with dementia [44]. The liaison mental health services have not only shown improved clinical outcomes as measured by the length of hospital stay or discharge to original residence but also suggested cost effective models. However, concerns have been raised about the reliability and validity of the various studies included in this systematic review [45]. The hospital liaison multidisciplinary mental health team is the model advised in the United Kingdom to offer a general hospital a complete service.

The Rapid Assessment Interface and Discharge (RAID) service model is an example in the United Kingdom where a psychiatry liaison service provides MDT input to acutely unwell older people with existing mental health admitted to hospital [46]. The RAID service has shown to be an effective, enhanced service model for older people who are at risk for dementia or other mental health problems and has shown good outcomes with quality improvements in the care of older people [46].

Collateral history from the family or carers remains the key feature for initial assessment. If dementia is suspected in a person, a full medical assessment must be completed, an example being the British Geriatrics Society's guidance on CGA of the frail older people [12]. Older people in the hospitals should be assessed for mood, anxiety and depression. The hospital anxiety and depression scale (HADS) is a simple, valid and reliable tool for use in hospital practice [47]. It is a self-assessment screening tool, which warrants further assessment based on abnormal scores. The score for the entire scale for emotional distress can range from 0 to 42, with higher scores indicating more distress. Score for each subscale (anxiety and depression) can range from 0 to 21 (normal 0–7, mild 8–10, moderate 11–14, severe 15–21) [48]. A short-form Geriatric Depression Scale (GDS) consisting of 15 questions can be used for depression [49]. Any positive score above 5 on the GDS short form should prompt a detailed assessment and evaluation. Generalised anxiety disorder (GAD) is the most common mental disorder encountered in older patients and is often accompanied by depression. It could be helpful to assess older person's emotional state and sense of well-being as they may report psychological burden of the disease, for example, fear of falling or fear of being in the hospital which is associated with loss of independence by older people. History of delusions and hallucinations or previous use of psychotropic drugs may suggest a mental health problem. Patient's permission should be sought before interviewing their relatives or carers for collateral history.

Following initial suspicion or diagnosis of a mental health problem in older people, a more collaborative work between physicians and old age psychiatrists for the prompt diagnosis and management of mental health problems will improve outcome [46].

2.3. Drugs

Drug prescribing increases with both age and incidence of co-morbidities [50, 51]. Polypharmacy is defined as use of either five or more concurrent medications or, at least, one potentially inappropriate drug. Half of older people aged between 65 and 74 years and two-thirds of those aged 75 years and over are affected by polypharmacy including conventional and complementary medicines [52]. Polypharmacy is associated with adverse outcomes including hospital admissions, falls, delirium, cognitive impairment and mortality [53, 54]. Although drugs have an important role in managing co-morbidities, it is not without harm and adverse outcomes [55].

There is conflicting evidence that psychotropic medications are associated with higher falls in people with dementia [56, 57] though there is clear evidence that there is associated increased fall risk in cognitively intact people [58]. Other classes of drugs including Parkinson's disease drugs, anticonvulsants, steroids and fluoroquinolone can result in acute confusion [59]. Drug interactions could impair electrolytes, cause postural hypotension, hypothermia, gait disorder or gastrointestinal disturbance, resulting in prolonged hospital admission [55].

Therefore, all older inpatients should have drug review and withdrawal of any possible offending agent if practical would be logical. This can be based on screening tool of older persons' prescriptions (STOPP), and a tool to alert doctors to commence appropriate treatment (START) criteria should be used [60]. Patients should also be assessed for their ability to manage their drugs, understanding of drug, dexterity and vision. At the same time, appropriate new medications if deemed necessary and evidence-based should be commenced. Older people with cognitive impairment should be prescribed with greater care, adhering to the principle of, 'starting low and going slow' [61].

2.4. Physical performance

Gait and balance are regulated by both central and peripheral nervous system; thus, various neurological disorders can result in postural instability and poor mobility. Balance system can be affected by the impact of neurological disease on postural responses, postural tone, sensory feedback, visuospatial disorder, executive dysfunction or delayed latencies. Gait disorders have been classified into lower (e.g. peripheral), middle (e.g. spinal, basal ganglia) and higher level gait disorders (e.g. frontal or psychogenic) [62]. The more pragmatic approach could be used to describe gait disorders including hypokinetic gait disorders, dystonic, hemi- or paraparetic gait, ataxia, vestibular, neuromuscular and psychogenic gait [62]. All components of gait including initiation of walking, step length, coordination, walking speed, symmetry, stride width, rhythm and posture should be assessed. Various tools/scales can be used for further assessment of gait and balance (**Table 3**). Most physicians work closely with PT and rely on their assessment of patient's needs in relation to mobility, balance and posture. Multidimensional assessment and multiagency management of mobility in older people lead to better outcomes.

	Technique	Normal values
Turn 180° [63]	A measure of dynamic postural stability, asking a patient to take few steps and then turn around by 180° to face opposite direction. Count the number of steps taken to complete a 180° turn	Five or less steps
3-m TUG test [64]	A measurement of mobility. A person is asked to stand up from seated position, walk for 3 m, turn and walk back to a chair and sit down. Measure the time taken in seconds	12 or fewer seconds, can vary with age by 2–4 s
Near tandem stand [65]	A measure of balance and ankle strength. A person is asked to stand in a near tandem position with their bare feet separated laterally by 2.5 cm with the heel of the front foot 2.5 cm anterior to the great toe of the back with their eyes closed. A person can hold arms out or move the body to help keep the balance but do not move the feet	Able to stand >30 s with eyes closed
Alternate step test [66]	A measure of strength, balance, coordination and stair climbing. It provides a measure of mediolateral stability. A person should be asked to place alternate whole left and right bare foot onto a 19-cm high stepper for a total of eight times	10 or fewer seconds, can vary with age by 2–4 s
Sit-to-stand test [67]	A measurement of functional mobility, balance and lower limb strength. A person should be able to stand up and sit down five times with crossed arms from a 45-cm straight-backed chair	11.4 s (60–69 years); 12.6 s (70–79 years); 14.8 s (80–89 years)

Table 3. Gait and balance assessment tools.

Physical activity interventions for people with an intact cognition are well documented and shown to be effective in improving balance and reducing falls. People with dementia are two to three times more likely to fall [16] and risk is further increased in people with Lewy body dementia (LBD) and Parkinson's disease dementia (PDD) [23, 68]. There is limited evidence showing significant gait and balance improvement following the targeted exercise programme in the community-dwelling older people with dementia [69]. More recently, it has been shown that supervise exercise training in people with dementia living in community could improve muscle strength and physical activity [70]. There is dearth of similar studies in the hospital setting and further research is required. A simple flexible home-based muscle strengthening and balance-training exercise programme along with medication could improve the physical performance in the older people.

2.5. Functional status

It is not uncommon for older people to be admitted to the hospital with functional deterioration or increased dependence, thus unable to cope. Older people admitted to the hospital with an acute medical problem, 'geriatric giants' [71, 72], incontinence, immobility, postural instability (falls) and intellectual impairment (dementia) or who are frail with one or more disability should get an appropriate functional assessment. A typical geriatric assessment for such people should begin with a review of their functional status. This is usually captured in two commonly used functional status measurement—basic ADL and instrumental ADL (IADL). The ADL that is initially affected includes complex or IADLs such as shopping, handling finances, driving, cooking or using the telephone followed by basic ADL including bathing, dressing, toileting, transferring, continence or feeding. Whether patients can function independently or need some help is usually determined by OT, as part of the comprehensive geriatric assessment. OTs work closely with the physiotherapists to assess patient's own environmental and home status with the identification of appropriate equipment and its delivery before discharge. In addition to optimising functional independence, OT intervention also enhances home comfort, safe use of available facilities, safe access to transport or potential use of telehealth technology and local resources.

The assessment of functional limitations is best completed by an interview with the person and caregiver with open-ended questions about their ability to perform activities. They can further be assessed by direct observation either in their usual place of residence or whilst performing a routine activity, for example, toilet use. The functional status can also be assessed using a standardised assessment instrument with questions about specific ADLs and IADLs. There are more than 15 validated scales to complete functional assessments including Katz index of independence in activities of daily living [73], the modified Blessed dementia scale [74], the instrumental activities of daily living scale [75], the Functional Assessment Questionnaire [76], Functional Assessment Staging Test [77], Barthel Activities of Daily Living Index Scale [78], Alzheimer's Disease Co-operative Study-Activities of Daily Living Inventory [79], Disability Assessment for Dementia [80] and Bristol activities of daily living [81].

The functional scales can detect early functional impairment and often help discriminate mild dementia in comparison to those with no cognitive impairment. The scales that assess complex social functional activities are better in detecting dementia compared to those scales that involve basic ADLs [82]. A good timely recognition of functional difficulties may arrest further decline, postponing the need for care-home placement. The functional assessment scales can only provide a guidance and these scales are commonly used to assess the treatment efficacy in scientific research studies.

2.6. Continence assessment

Urinary incontinence (UI) is defined by the International Continence Society as 'the complaint of any involuntary leakage of urine'. Older people may assume that UI is a normal consequence of ageing and often may not be reported. UI is a common problem and older people may feel embarrassed to discuss the problem and avoid evaluation. Incontinence is associated with social isolation, institutionalisation and medical complication including skin irritation, pressure sores, recurrent infections and falls. The prevalence of urinary incontinence depends on the age and gender; for older women, the estimated prevalence of urinary incontinence ranges from 17 to 55% (median = 35%, mean = 34%). In comparison, incontinence prevalence for older men ranges from 11 to 34% (median = 17%, mean = 22%) [83].

There is a strong association of faecal incontinence (FI) with age; FI increases from 2.6% in 20–29-year-old up to 15.3% in 70 years or above [84]. In hospital settings, UI can be an atypical presentation and is a risk factor for adverse outcomes. The aetiology of incontinence in older people is often multifactorial. People with cognitive impairment usually encounter UI and later FI. Older people often find it difficult and challenging to express the need of regular toilet use, and as dementia progresses, it could be difficult to identify toilet or use it appropriately. Incontinence and inability to use toilet independently can be frustrating and distressing, which may lead to psychological burden, isolation, immobility or institutionalisation.

Therefore, a good continence assessment should be an essential component for any older people admitted to hospital to ensure good-quality person-centred care, promoting independent living. Assessment of precipitating factors and identification of treatable, potentially reversible conditions are essential steps. Continence problems can be secondary to drug side effects, constipation, impaired mobility, arthritic pain, inappropriate clothing or dexterity.

A good clinical history could categorise UI as stress UI (involuntary urine leakage on exertion), urgency UI (a sudden compelling desire to urinate) or mixed UI (involuntary urine leakage associated with both urgency and exertion). Overactive bladder (OAB) is defined as urgency that occurs with or without incontinence and usually with frequency and nocturia. Bladder diary (72-h urine frequency volume chart) and pre- and post-void bladder scan support clinical diagnosis. Vaginal inspection is helpful to exclude vaginal atrophy, prolapse or infections. Older people with FI should have an anorectal examination to exclude faecal loading, lower gastrointestinal cancer, rectal prolapse, anal sphincter problems or haemorrhoids. Neurological causes of cauda equina syndrome, frontal lobe tumours, neurodegenerative disorders or stroke could also result in UI or FI.

The continence problems can be minimised by promoting regular toilet use, appropriate toilet adaptations and providing walking aids to improve accessibility to toilet. Nocturnal incontinence remains a challenging situation but can be managed using various containment methods or limiting fluid intake in the evening. Drug treatment after specialist continence assessment is usually the next step if non-drug measures failed to provide symptomatic benefits. The aim should be to treat the underlying cause but people who continue to have episodes of UI or FI after initial management should be considered for specialised management.

2.7. Nutritional assessment

Older people admitted with an acute illness are at increased risk of weight loss and this remains a challenge for the teams in the hospital setting. Acute illness can result in loss of appetite, and management of an acute illness may take priority, therefore making older people more vulnerable in the hospitals, particularly those with cognitive impairment or those who cannot communicate their needs. The National UK Dementia Audit Report in 2013 showed that nutritional assessments were undertaken in less than 10% of patients in some hospitals [85].

A detailed nutritional assessment should be undertaken on admission to hospital and should include any recent weight loss, dietary intake and habits. The risk factors including dry mouth, poor oral hygiene, problems with dexterity, reduced vision, acute or chronic confusion, constipation or pain should be explored and actively managed to avoid poor nutrition. Regular nutritional assessments using Malnutrition Universal Screening Tool (MUST) can be helpful and this has been validated to be used by any health professional in the hospital. It is a five-step screening tool, which can identify those who are at risk of weight loss or are malnourished [86].

A collective and simple approach with involvement of family and carers can prevent malnutrition during hospitalisation. Patients should be offered small frequent meals and regular snacks or preferred food is often helpful. Protected meal times and regular prompting or assistance for those with cognitive impairment can lead to improved food intake [87].

2.8. Personal hygiene

2.8.1. Oral and dental hygiene

Higher levels of poor oral health can be commonly observed and it is challenging to provide good and regular oral hygiene care to older people in hospitals. The oral hygiene in older people can be compromised secondary to impaired sensory functions, reduced physical dexterity and functional dependence. Older people are often on polypharmacy including anticholinergics, diuretics, antidepressants and antipsychotics. The common side effects of drugs are reduced salivary flow, which could affect the efficiency of chewing, leading to dental problems. Older people with cognitive deficits are at higher risk of developing oral diseases and conditions including dental caries, dental plaques and missing teeth [84]. Poor oral hygiene can also be related to uncontrolled diabetes, inappropriately fitted dentures, lack of teeth, poor mobility or salivary gland dysfunction [88].

Oral Health Assessment Tool (OHAT) screening has been proposed for the timely assessment of oral and dental hygiene. This tool has been validated for use by nursing staff in care-home residents [89] also those with dementia [90]. There could be reluctance and resistivity to maintain basic good oral hygiene by choice or lack of knowledge/information. Enhanced engagement of carers with oral hygiene strategies, a good education on oral hygiene in older people and timely identification of oral health problems by regular dental consultations could be effective in preventing oral diseases.

2.8.2. Skin

Older people, in general, are at higher risk of skin problems including pruritus, eczematous dermatitis, purpura, venous insufficiency and pressure ulcers. Other risk factors include loss of protective fat, malnutrition, frailty, sarcopenia, urinary or bowel incontinence and cognitive impairment. The risk of pressure ulcers further increases with hospitalisation secondary to poor oral intake and reduced physical activities.

Prompt assessment and appropriate skin-care plan including good personal hygiene, healthy balanced diet, avoiding excessive heat and friction, promoting continence and early mobilisation are the key factors to minimise the risk of skin breakdown.

http://dx.doi.org/10.5772/64294

2.9. Vision

Visual impairment is common in older people and this risk increases with advancing age. The visual impairment increases from 6.2% at ages 75–79 to 36.9% at age 90 or over [91]. Blindness also increases from 0.6 (75–79) to 6.9% in 90 years or over. Visual impairment in older people is often under-diagnosed and can complicate the accurate assessment of ADLs. Older people who experience visual problems may avoid activities that require good vision and become isolated or even need to be institutionalised. People with cognitive impairment may further experience visuoperceptual difficulties such as visual hallucinations, colour perception, background contrast and depth perception.

Simple measures such as the use of blinds or shades to reduce glare, wearing the correct glasses, minimising visual and physical obstacles, using colours and contrasts to mark different areas, assistive technologies such as automatic lights, audio labels or audio books can minimise the risks. Requesting eyesight testing by involving optometrists or ophthalmologists to examine eyes for the causes of sight loss is a first step in defining appropriate interventions.

2.10. Hearing

Hearing impairment is one of the three most common chronic diseases along with arthritis and hypertension [92]. People with hearing loss are less likely to participate in social activities and are less satisfied with their life as a whole. Hearing loss does not only affect individual's emotional well-being but also their ability to manage IADLs. Older people with hearing loss are prone to develop dementia [93] and hearing loss is commonly reported in people with dementia.

Hearing loss can be conductive and sensorineural. The causal factors that may contribute to hearing impairment could include ear wax build-up, ear infections, degenerative ageing process, excess occupational noise, stroke, head injuries, drug side effects or neoplasms like an acoustic neuroma.

All patients with hearing impairment require thorough examination and presence of dementia should not preclude assessment for a hearing aid. Simple measures such as speaking in a normal tone, giving attention and making eye contact are helpful. Appropriate seating, eliminating background noise and repeating the key phrases or summary points improve communication. Hearing aids are often useful, though they do not improve cognitive function or reduce BPSD but has shown that patients improved on global measures of change [94].

2.11. Pain

Pain should be treated as a fifth vital sign. Pain assessment involves holistic evaluation of the person on the first presentation of pain and then following up with regular pain assessment. Pain assessment should include the site of pain, type, precipitating factors and impact of pain on the individual. Physical assessment should be performed for any skin bruise or infection, constipation, reduced range of joint movement, vertebral tenderness, recent injury or fracture. There are several pain scales available, visual analogue scale or the numerical rating scales are most useful.

Older people with cognitive impairment and those who cannot verbally communicate their symptoms particularly pain, observation or collateral information from relative or carer or suggestion of change in person's behaviour could help to assess the severity of pain [95]. The numeric pain-rating scale (0–10, where 10 being most severe pain) is often used in routine clinical practice. The specific pain-screening tools such as 'Assessment of Discomfort in Dementia (ADD)' are available to be used in patients with cognitive impairment. The tool involves assessing pain history, physical examination and administration of analgesics and giving analgesics as needed [96].

2.12. Sociocultural assessment

It is important to assess person's language, ethnic background, cultural beliefs, personality, education, family experience, socio-economic status and life experience to complete assessment holistically and provide person-centred care. A detailed assessment of social network, daytime activities and informal support available from family or friends should be done on the first day of admission to the hospital.

A prompt, patient-centred identification of the requirement of social services input helps with safe timely discharge to the most suitable and friendly environment. Social Worker (SW) should ideally be allocated if a need for social services is anticipated at the time of hospital admission. Once all the needs of the patient are identified, SW should be contacted to organise formal carers or care-home placement if the patient is not suitable for home discharge.

2.13. Quality of life

The quality of life (QoL) assessment was almost unknown 20 years ago but it is now an established fact that the psychological burden of an illness cannot be described fully by measures of disease status. It has been acknowledged that various psychosocial factors such as apprehension, anxiety, restricted mobility, difficulty in fulfilling ADLs and the financial burden must also be addressed to complete holistic assessment of older people. The most important constituents of the quality of life in older age from older people's perspective are having good social relationships with family, friends and neighbours; participating in social and voluntary activities and individual interests and having good health and functional ability [93, 94]. Other measures of good QoL include living in a good home and neighbourhood, having a positive outlook and psychological well-being, having an adequate income and maintaining independence and control over one's life [97, 98].

The assessment of a patient's experience of disease and its effect on their quality and outcome framework (QoF) should be one of the central components of healthcare assessment to acknowledge safe and early hospital discharge. The family members should be involved on occasions when it is difficult to measure the patient's QoL due to underlying cognitive impairments and communication deficits [99].

2.14. Sexuality

Sexual desires and the physical capacity to engage in sex continue throughout life. Though many older people enjoy an active sex life, there has been a little mention of sexuality or the problems that older people may face related to sexual issues in government policies [96].

There are several causes for loss of interest and frequency of sexual activity in later life including physical health problems, emotional distress, drug use, male or female sexual dysfunction, practical problems, willingness or lack of partner and not necessarily only ageing [100]. Healthcare professionals routinely avoid discussing sexual problems with older people; however, sharing physical relations and closeness are very important in maintaining long-term emotional and physical intimacy.

3. Examination

Thorough physical examination from head to toe in a systematic fashion is essential, especially if the cause of acute illness or deterioration is not clear from the history. The clinical signs may not be very obvious as often older people have an atypical presentation, for example, hypothermia instead of hyperthermia, lack of typical signs of heart failure or meningism. Older people sometimes get fatigued after history taking; in such occasions, physical examination may have to be done at a different time.

4. Investigations

The investigations should be requested only as indicated by clinical examination. For example, urine analysis should only be done if symptomatic, unexplained systemic sepsis or delirium. As over diagnosis of urinary tract infection may point towards inadequate assessment of frail older people. The common investigations usually include blood oxygen saturation, complete blood count, kidney, liver, bone profile, urinalysis and a chest radiograph. An electrocardiogram should be obtained because there is a higher risk of silent myocardial infarction in older people. Other investigations including CT brain or lumbar puncture are helpful in those with unexplained altered mental status.

5. Management

The drug and non-drug treatment should be evidence based with aim to treat underlying medical illness. The management of older people needs close liaison work with geriatricians, acute physicians, ED and MDT. The model of care should be established in hospitals so that supportive care for older people can be provided within the first few hours of an admission [101]. For older people with frailty, multiple co-morbidities and an acute illness, admission should be to an Emergency Frailty Unit (EFU), a separate unit within an AMU. EFU or a similar unit led by a geriatrician and the multidisciplinary team (MDT) could not only provide comprehensive person-centred care but also enhance clinical outcomes irrespective of age [102]. In addition, a close working with liaison old-age psychiatry can improve outcome [43]. There should be minimal intra- and inter-hospital transfer to reduce the risk of delirium. Interventions should be planned very carefully and keeping the associated risks in mind, for example, older people should not be routinely catheterised unless there is evidence of urinary retention.

5.1. Patient education

Hospital admission could be a good opportunity to educate older people and their carers on chronic disease and its management, healthy lifestyles, physical activity, sufficient fluid intake and healthy nutritious foods. Alcohol consumption is under-recognised in older people and an informal discussion by a health professional could be beneficial. A brief discussion with a clinical pharmacist can improve adherence to medication in older people.

5.2. Staff training

Training in hospitals is usually directed towards patient safety, managing acute medical conditions, good handover, and rapid response to a sick patient; however, it is equally essential to augment knowledge and skills of hospital staff in assessing and managing older frail patients. The majority of older patients are admitted to hospital through AMU or directly to EFU, which justifies the need for an EFU geriatrician taking a lead in staff training at the front end [101]. Nursing staff need regular training and education on geriatric giants and frailty [103]. Systematic nurse training has shown to reduce work-related stress [104] and improved outcomes as measured by reduction of inpatient falls [105]. Dementia awareness training should be mandatory and should also be included in induction programmes. Staff members should be encouraged to collect personal information about people with dementia to help improve care, for example, use of 'This is Me' document. Information sharing and communication among staff, carers and patients should be improved to ensure that all staff coming into contact with older frail people are aware of their problems and associated needs.

5.3. Caregiver problems

Occasionally, problems of older patients are related to neglect or abuse by their caregiver. Hospital staff should consider the possibility of 'elder abuse' if there are suggestions on clinical assessment. Certain injury patterns are particularly suggestive, including frequent bruising (middle of the back, upper arms or groin area), fearfulness of a caregiver or unexplained burns.

5.4. Service outcome review

The regular involvements in audits and analysis of hospital readmission rates, delayed discharge and mortality could identify the needs for service improvement and provision of safe enhanced good quality care for older people.

6. Discharge planning

Older people admitted to hospital are entitled to receive a smooth transition from one stage of hospital care to the next stage of care in the community. A lack of coordinated and person-centred discharge planning can lead to poor outcomes for the patients, thus affecting their health and safety. Poor discharge planning can also lead to inappropriate prolonged LoS or premature discharge and thus result in possible readmission to the hospital.

6.1. Independence

Maintenance of independence and participation in social and voluntary activities are the key benefits of home discharge. This has been quoted as one of the major elements of good QoL. Older people usually have a fear of losing independence as a result of ageing. Older people have reported that being independent, free to please oneself and freedom from time constraints are the best things about growing old [106]. Independence is usually associated with good health, living in own home and ability to walk independently. However, independence is felt to be lost if older people are unable to manage their ADLs. The perceived physical environmental barriers and mobility or ADLs have significant positive correlation [107].

6.2. Safe, effective and timely discharge

The principal aims of the safe and effective discharge process are to ensure that patients should not stay in the hospital any longer than necessary. Discharge should be on 'pull system' rather than on 'push system' in order to maximise their social interaction and independence by providing timely and comprehensive carer support according to their needs.

Discharge planning should be a systematic coordinated process, which should begin on the first contact with health professional based on the specific needs of the patient with documentation of expected date of discharge (EDD). An older person must be assumed to have capacity unless suggested otherwise and all patients should be encouraged to take their informed decision with an aim to maintain their maximum independence and social interaction in the community.

Where a discharge process is complex, a safe discharge meeting (SDM) should be set and should be attended by members of MDT with SW and preferably by the patient's relative/carer. There should be a clear purpose of the meeting and needs of the patients should be discussed. The information should be gathered from the SW regarding existing care support services. If there is no need for further specialist referral then discharge date should be set and appropriate requirement of support should be requested by involving social services or voluntary organisations. The confirmation of fitness to discharge must be agreed at least 24 h in advance of EDD with appropriate arrangements for transport.

6.3. Ethical issues related to discharge

The patient's autonomy should be respected both ethically and legally considering that a patient can understand proposed place of discharge, alternatives, risks and benefits in order to consent or refuse it. Patient's autonomy also requires consulting them and obtaining their informed consent before planning a discharge. The healthcare professionals should practice the principles of beneficence and non-maleficence together and aim at producing net medical benefit with minimal or no harm

6.4. Individual's interests and family wishes

The patient's interests and wishes should be taken into account when considering discharge planning and future care. The hospitalised patients can wax and wane in the level of alertness, so they should be assessed when they are fully awake and have not received any medications, which can impair their cognitive functions. If there are any doubts about the patient's expressed wishes, they should be evaluated at a later stage. There should be an attempt to involve the family and carers to organise patient-centred hospital discharge process, particularly for those patients who have underlying cognitive or uncorrected sensory impairment.

6.5. Decision-making capacity

According to English Law, an adult has the right to make decisions affecting his or her own life, whether the reasons for that choice are rational, irrational, unknown or even non-existent. Adults over 16 or those who lack capacity to make their own decisions to medical care and treatment are protected by The Mental Capacity Act (MCA) (UK).

The MCA provides a statutory framework and aims to support an individual's right to protect them from any harm caused due to lack of capacity to make autonomous decisions for themselves [108]. Therefore, every effort should be made to support people who lack capacity to make their own decisions; however, if the person clearly lacks capacity, this should be formally assessed. The decision should be discussed among MDT members and 'best interest meetings' should be organised in liaison with family or carers to make important decisions.

7. Follow-up

Older people discharged should have appropriate access to outpatient follow-up clinics, intermediate and social-care services. There should be effective electronic information-sharing with primary care and community.

7.1. End-of-life care

Some older frail people discharged from hospital could have a poor outcome. Mortality rates for frail older people in the year following discharge from AMUs are high (26% in one series) [109]. Most very old individuals with severe dementia in the community die away from a usual place of residence and hospitals remain the most common place of death [110]. Dementia care during end of life is not similar to the other life-limiting illness [111]. The symptoms experienced by the people with dementia are similar to those with cancer patients but often dementia is not considered as a life-threatening illness. People with dementia not only experience symptoms over longer period but also need more support from the social services and palliative teams [112].

Therefore, healthcare and social care professionals should discuss and record advance care planning statements, advance decisions to refuse particular treatments or preferred place of care in future. The decisions made should be shared with community team and families/carers.

8. Current evidence on CGA

The concept of CGA evolved as a result of multiple complex problems in older patients. The first comprehensive meta-analysis of the benefits of CGA was conducted in 1993, which demonstrated that CGA could improve the functional status, survival, reduce the hospital LoS and subsequent health service contacts as well as reduce care-home admissions. This meta-analysis also showed that an improvement in physical function from the geriatric evaluation and management unit (GEMU) interventions was maintained at 12 months (odds ratio (OR): 1.72; 95% confidence interval (CI): 1.06–2.80) [113].

Although there is a proven role for intensive geriatric rehabilitation in improving the functional outcome and independence in patients with hip fracture [114, 115], other randomised control trials (RCTs) comparing CGA to routine care in later years showed no significance in physical functioning or hospital LoS [116–118].

The systematic review of the literature including 20 randomised controlled trials (RCT) (10, 427 participants) of inpatient CGA for a mixed elderly inpatient population was conducted in 2005. This review confirmed the benefits of inpatient CGA and increased chances of living at home at 1 year, and improved physical and cognitive function with no long-term mortality benefits [119]. More recently, systematic review and meta-analysis involving 17 trials with 4780 people compared the effects of general or orthopaedic geriatric rehabilitation programmes with usual care. The specifically designed inpatient rehabilitation for geriatric patients showed beneficial effects over usual care for functional improvement, preventing admissions to nursing homes and reducing mortality [120].

It appears that setting up a CGA unit carries increased staffing costs or insufficient cost-effective data are available [120] but in American studies of medical and surgical patients the financial costs of managing care for older people in a specialised hospital unit were not more expensive than caring for patients on a usual-care ward [121, 122]. A meta-analysis of RCTs in 2011 has confirmed not only benefits of CGA but also a potential cost reduction compared to general medical care [123]. However, the nature of CGA varies and many, but not all, older people have complex care needs. Therefore, it is difficult to identify which patients will benefit the most and those at risk of adverse outcomes. Frailty status measurement by an index of accumulated deficits generated from routine CGA has shown strong association with adverse outcome; therefore, frailty index may have clinical utility, augmenting clinical judgement in the management of older inpatients [39]. In summary, older frail patients should have early access to inpatient CGA and interdisciplinary involvement in a specialist ward for optimal care to reduce LoS, regain function and physical stability [120].

9. Limitations to a good assessment

1. Lack of training for doctors, nurses and multidisciplinary members and unfamiliarity with key principles and practices of geriatric medicine [103, 124].
2. Awareness and support to MDT members is relatively poor.
3. Lack of interest and associated negative societal attitudes towards older people.
4. Limited access to dementia care training to meet the complex care needs of older people [125].

10. Conclusion

Comprehensive geriatric assessment has proven benefit and this should be considered as the evidence-based standard of care for the frail older inpatients. There is a need to configure emergency, acute medical and geriatric services to deliver high-quality CGA for frail older people at the earliest possible time following contact with the acute sector. The aim should be better integration among multidisciplinary members to achieve well-coordinated, high standard of care and improve outcomes. Older people are the major users of acute care and AMU is the key area for initial decision-making; therefore, staff training to meet the needs of frail older people in Acute Medical Unit or Emergency Frailty Unit is mandatory.

11. Conflict of interest

The author has no financial or any other kind of personal conflicts with this article.

Acknowledgements

The author like to thank all members of the Department of Geriatric Medicine, Ysbyty Ystrad Fawr (ABUHB), for their continued support for research activities. The author also like to express his appreciation to Miss Salma Zabaneh, Education Centre/Library, for her support.

http://dx.doi.org/10.5772/64294

Author details

Inderpal Singh

Address all correspondence to: inder.singh@wales.nhs.uk

Department of Geriatric Medicine, Ysbyty Ystrad Fawr, Aneurin Bevan University Health Board, Wales, UK

References

[1] Hospitals on the edge? The time for action. A report by the Royal College of Physicians September 2012. Available at: https://www.rcplondon.ac.uk/guidelines-policy/hospitals-edge-time-action Accessed on April 24, 2016.

[2] Rubenstein LZ, Stuck AE, Siu AL, Wieland D. Impact of geriatric evaluation and management programs on defined outcomes: overview of the evidence. J Am Geriatr Soc 1991; 39: 8–16S.

[3] Covinsky KE, Palmer RM, Fortinsky RH et al. Loss of independence in activities of daily living in older adults hospitalized with medical illnesses: increased vulnerability with age. J Am Geriatr Soc 2003; 51: 451–8.

[4] Mahoney JE, Sager MA, Jalaluddin M. New walking dependence associated with hospitalisation for acute medical illness: incidence and significance. J Gerontol A Biol Sci Med Sci 1998; 53(4): 307–12.

[5] Mudge AM, O'Rourke P, Denaro CP. Timing and risk factors for functional changes associated with medical hospitalization in older patients. J Gerontol A Biol Sci Med Sci 2010; 65: 866–72.

[6] Sager MA, Franke T, Inouye SK et al. Functional outcomes of acute medical illness and hospitalization in older persons. Arch Intern Med 1996; 156(6): 645–52.

[7] Roland M and Abel G. Reducing emergency admissions: are we on the right track? BMJ 2012; 345:e6017.

[8] Scott I. Optimising care of the hospitalised elderly - a literature review and suggestions for future research. Aust N Z J Med 1999; 29(2): 254–64.

[9] Cheitlin MD. Cardiovascular physiology-changes with aging. Am J Geriatr Cardiol 2003; 12(1): 9–13.

[10] Sharma G and Goodwin J. Effect of aging on respiratory system physiology and immunology. Clin Interv Aging 2006; 1(3): 253–60.

[11] Rockwood K, Rockwood MR, Mitnitski A. Physiological redundancy in older adults in relation to the change with age in the slope of a frailty index. Am Geriatr Soc 2010; 58(2): 318–23.

[12] British Geriatrics Society (2010). Comprehensive assessment of the frail older patient. Available at: http://www.bgs.org.uk/index.php/topresources/publicationfind/good-practice/195-gpgcgassessment Accessed on April 24, 2016

[13] Lamb SE, Jorstad-Stein EC, Hauer K et al: Development of a common outcome data set for fall injury prevention trials: the prevention of falls network Europe consensus. J Am Geriatr Soc 2005; 53: 1618–22.

[14] Talbot LA, Musiol RJ, Witham EK, Metter EJ. Falls in young, middle-aged and older community dwelling adults: perceived cause, environmental factors and injury. BMC Public Health 2005; 5: 86.

[15] Masud T, Morris R. Epidemiology of falls. Age Aging 2001; 30–54: 3–7.

[16] Tinetti ME, Speechley M, Ginter SF. Risk factors for falls among elderly persons living within the community. N Eng J Med 1988; 319: 1701–7.

[17] Close J, Ellis M, Hooper R, Glucksman E, Jackson S, Swift C. Prevention of falls in the elderly trial (PROFET): a randomised controlled trial. Lancet 1999; 353: 93–7.

[18] Schwendimann R, Bühler H, De Geest S, Milisen K. Characteristics of hospital inpatient falls across clinical departments. Gerontology 2008; 54(6): 342–8.

[19] Singh I, Okeke J. Risk of inpatient falls is increased with single rooms. BMJ 2013; 347: f6344.

[20] Sattin RW, Lambert Huber DA, DeVito CA, et al. The incidence of fall injury events among the elderly in a defined population. Am J Epidemiol 1990; 131: 1028–37.

[21] Singh I, Okeke J, Edwards C. Outcome of in-patient falls in hospitals with 100% single rooms and multi-bedded wards. Age Ageing 2015; 44 (6): 1032–5.

[22] Roche JJW, Wenn RT, Sahota O, Moran CG. Effect of comorbidities and postoperative complications on mortality after hip fracture in elderly people: prospective observational cohort study. BMJ. 2005; 331: 1374.

[23] Ballard CG, Shaw F, Lowery K, Mckeith I, Kenny R. The prevalence, assessment and associations of falls in dementia with Lewy bodies and Alzheimer's disease. Dement Geriatr Cogn Disord. 1999; 10(2): 97–103.

[24] Singh I. Approach to Falls in the Young, Middle Aged, and the Elderly. In: Sudesh Prabhakar, Gagandeep Singh, Differential Diagnosis in Neurology, Edition: 1/e. Jaypee Brothers Medical Publishers, pp. 281–6.

[25] Task Force on DSM-IV. Diagnostic and statistical manual of mental disorders. 4th edition. Text revision (DSM-IV-TR). American Psychiatric Association, Washington DC, 2000.

[26] Inouye SK, van Dyck CH, Alessi CA, Balkin S, Siegal A, Horwitz RI. Clarifying confusion: the confusion assessment method. Ann Intern Med 1990; 15; 113(12): 941–8.

[27] Fong TG, Jones RN, Marcantonio ER, et al. Adverse outcomes after hospitalization and delirium in persons with Alzheimer disease. Ann Intern Med 2012; 156(12): 848–56.

[28] Siddiqi N, House AO, Holmes JD. Occurrence and outcome of delirium in medical inpatients: a systematic literature review. Age Ageing 2006; 35(4): 350–364.

[29] Andrew MK, Freter SH, Rockwood K. Incomplete functional recovery after delirium in elderly people: a prospective cohort study. BMC Geriatr 2005; 5: 5. doi:10.1186/1471–2318-5–5

[30] Sampson EL, Blanchard MR, Jones L, Tookman A, King M. Dementia in the acute hospital: prospective cohort study of prevalence and mortality. Br J Psychiatry 2009; 195: 61–6.

[31] Singh I, Edwards C, Okeke J. Impact of cognitive impairment on inpatient falls in single room setting and its adverse outcomes. J Gerontol Geriatr Res. 2015; S4: S4–001. doi: 10.4172/2167–7182.S4–001

[32] Marengoni A, Nobili A, Romano V, et al. Adverse clinical events and mortality during hospitalization and 3 months after discharge in cognitively impaired elderly patients. J Gerontol A Biol Sci Med Sci 2013; 68(4): 419–25.

[33] Singh I, Varanasi A, Williamson K. Assessment and management of dementia in the general hospital setting. Rev Clin Gerontol 2014; 24: 1–14.

[34] Fried LP, Tangen CM, Walston J, et al. Cardiovascular Health Study Collaborative Research Group. Frailty in older adults: evidence for a phenotype. J Gerontol Med Sci 2001; 56: 146–56.

[35] Rockwood K, Mitnitski A. Frailty in relation to the accumulation of deficits. J Gerontol Med Sci 2007; 62: 722–7.

[36] Searle SD, Mitnitski A, Gahbauer EA, Gill TM, Rockwood K. A standard procedure for creating a frailty index. BMC Geriatr 2008; 8: 24.

[37] Jones D, Song X, Mitnitski A, Rockwood K. Evaluation of a frailty index based on a comprehensive geriatric assessment in a population based study of elderly Canadians. Aging Clin Exp Res 2005; 17: 465–71.

[38] Jones DM, Song X, Rockwood K. Operationalizing a frailty index from a standardized comprehensive geriatric assessment. J Am Geriatr Soc 2004; 52: 1929–33.

[39] Singh I, Gallacher J, Davis K, Johansen A, Eeles E, Hubbard RE. Predictors of adverse outcomes on an acute geriatric rehabilitation ward. Age Ageing 2012; 41: 242–6.

[40] Naylor C, Parsonage M, McDaid D, Knapp M, Fossey M, Galea A. Long-term conditions and mental health: the cost of co-morbidities. The King's Fund and Centre for Mental Health 2012. Available at: http://www.kingsfund.org.uk/sites/files/kf/field/field_publication_file/long-term-conditions-mental-health-cost-comorbidities-naylor-feb12.pdf. Accessed April 24, 2016.

[41] Weimer DL, Sager MA. Early identification and treatment of Alzheimer's disease: social and fiscal outcomes. Alzheimers Dement 2009; 5(3): 215–26.

[42] Blazer DG. Depression in late life: review and commentary. J Gerontol A Biol Sci Med Sci 2003; 58(3): 249–65.

[43] Singh I, Ramakrishna S, Williamson K. The rapid assessment interface and discharge service and its implications for patients with dementia. Clin Interv Aging 2013; 8:1101–8.

[44] Department of Health. National Service Framework for Older People. London: Department of Health; 2001 [Mar 2001]. Available from: https://www.gov.uk/government/uploads/system/uploads/attachment_data/file/198033/National_Service_Framework_for_Older_People.pdf. Accessed April 24, 2016.

[45] Holmes J, Montaňa C, Powell G, et al. Liaison Mental Health Services for Older People: A Literature Review, Service Mapping and In-depth Evaluation of Service Models. London: National Institute for Health Research Service Delivery and Organisation programme, Service Delivery and Organisation Programme; 2010 [Jun 2010]. Available at: http://www.nets.nihr.ac.uk/__data/assets/pdf_file/0016/81412/ES-08–1504-100.pdf. Accessed April 24, 2016.

[46] Tadros G, Salama RA, Kingston P, et al. Impact of an integrated rapid response psychiatric liaison team on quality improvement and cost savings: the Birmingham RAID model. Psychiatrist 2013; 37: 4–10.

[47] Snaith RP. The hospital anxiety and depression scale. Health Qual Life Outcomes 2003; 1: 29.

[48] Zigmond AS, Snaith RP. The hospital anxiety and depression scale. Acta Psychiatrica Scandinavica 1983; 67(6): 361–70.

[49] Greenberg SA. How to try this: the geriatric depression scale: short form. Am J Nurs 2007; 107(10): 60–9.

[50] Woodhouse K. Treating older people. Eur J Clin Pharmacol 2013; 69(1): 53–7.

[51] Ramage-Morin PL. Medication use among senior Canadians. Health Rep 2009; 20(1): 37–44.

[52] Morgan TK, Williamson M, Pirotta M, Stewart K, Myers SP, Barnes J. A national census of medicines use: a 24-hour snapshot of Australians aged 50 years and older. Med J Aust 2012; 16;196(1): 50–3.

[53] Hilmer SN, Gnjidic D. The effects of polypharmacy in older adults. Clin Pharmacol Ther 2009; 85: 86–8.

[54] Jyrkkä J, Enlund H, Korhonen MJ, Sulkava R, Hartikainen S. Polypharmacy status as an indicator of mortality in an elderly population. Drugs Aging 2009; 26(12): 1039–48.

[55] Mannesse CK, Derkx FH, de Ridder MA, Man in 't Veld AJ, van der Cammen TJ. Contribution of adverse drug reactions to hospital admission of older patients. Age Ageing 2000; 29(1): 35–9.

[56] Taylor ME, Lord SR, Delbaere K, Mikolaizak AS, Close JC. Physiological fall risk factors in cognitively impaired older people: a one year prospective study. Dement Geriatr Cogn Disord 2012; 34(3–4):181–9.

[57] Banerjee S. The use of antipsychotic medication for people with dementia: time for action. 2009 Available at: http://www.rcpsych.ac.uk/pdf/Antipsychotic%20Bannerjee %20Report.pdf. Accessed on April 24, 2016

[58] Hartikainen S, Lonnroos E, Louhivuori K. Medication as a risk factor for falls: critical systematic review. J Gerontol A Biol Sci Med Sci 2007; 62(10): 1172–81.

[59] von Moltke LL, Greenblatt DJ, Romach MK, Sellers EM. Cognitive toxicity of drugs used in the elderly. Dialogues Clin Neurosci 2001; 3(3): 181–90.

[60] Gallagher P, Baeyens J-P, Topinkova E, et al. Inter-rater reliability of STOPP (Screening Tool of Older Persons' Prescriptions) and START (Screening Tool to Alert doctors to Right Treatment) criteria amongst physicians in six European countries. Age Ageing 2009; 38(5): 603–6.

[61] Milton JC, Hill-Smith I, Jackson SHD. Prescribing for older people. BMJ. 2008;336: 606–9.

[62] Stolze H, Vieregge P, Deuschl G. Gait disturbances in neurology. Nervenarzt 2008; 79(4): 485–99.

[63] Nevitt MC, Cummings SR, Kidd S, et al. Risk factors for recurrent non-syncopal falls. A prospective study. JAMA 1989; 261(18): 2663–8.

[64] Podsiadlo D, Richardson S. The timed "Up & Go": a test of basic functional mobility for frail elderly persons. J Am Geriatr Soc 1991; 39: 142–8.

[65] Lord SR, Rogers MW, Howland A, Fitzpatrick R. Lateral stability, sensorimotor function and falls in older people. J Am Geriatr Soc 1999; 47(9): 1077–81.

[66] Berg KO, Wood-Dauphinee SL, Williams JI, Maki B. Measuring balance in the elderly: validation of an instrument. Can J Public Health 1992; 83: 7–11.

[67] Bohannon RW. Reference values for the five-repetition sit-to-stand test: a descriptive meta-analysis of data from elders. Percept Mot Skills 2006; 103(1): 215–22.

[68] Allan LM, Ballard CG, Rowan EN, Kenny RA. Incidence and prediction of falls in dementia: a prospective study in older people. PLoS One 2009, 4(5): e5521. doi:10.1371/journal.pone.0005521

[69] Suttanon P, Hill K, Said CM, Dodd KJ. Can balance exercise programmes improve balance and related physical performance measures in people with dementia. A systematic review. Eur Rev Aging Phys Act 2010; 7(1): 13–25.

[70] Hauer K, Schwenk M, Zieschang T, Essig M, Becker C, Oster P. Physical training improves motor performance in people with dementia: a randomized controlled trial. J Am Geriatr Soc 2012; 60(1): 8–15.

[71] Isaacs B. The challenge of geriatric medicine. Oxford University Press; 1992.

[72] Flacker JM. What is a geriatric syndrome anyway? Geriatrics Ageing 2003; 6(9): 58–9.

[73] Katz S, Ford AB, Moskowitz RW, Jackson BA, Jaffe MW. Studies of illness in the aged. The Index of ADL: a standardized measure of biological and psychosocial function. JAMA 1963; 185: 914–9.

[74] Erkinjuntti T, Hokkanen L, Sulkava R, Palo J. The blessed dementia scale as a screening test for dementia. Int J Geriat Psychiatry 1988; 3: 267–73.

[75] Lawton MP, Brody EM. "Assessment of older people: Self-maintaining and instrumental activities of daily living." Gerontologist 1969; 9: 179–86.

[76] Pfeffer RI, Kurosaki TT, Harrah CH, Chance JM, Filos S. Measurement of the functional activities in older adults in the community. J Geront 1982; 37: 323–9.

[77] Sclan SG, Reisberg B. Functional assessment staging (FAST) in Alzheimer's disease: reliability, validity, and ordinality. Int Psychogeriatr 1992; 4(1): 55–69.

[78] Mahoney FI, Barthel DW. Functional evaluation: the Barthel index. Md State Med J 1965; 14: 61–65.

[79] Galasko D, Bennet D, Sano M, et al. An inventory to assess activities of daily living for clinical trials in Alzheimer's disease. The Alzheimer's Disease Cooperative Study. Alzheimer Dis Assoc Disord 1997; 11: 33–9.

[80] Gélinas I, Gauthier L, McIntyre M, Gauthier S. Development of a functional measure for persons with Alzheimer's disease: the disability assessment for dementia. Am J Occup Ther 1999; 53: 471–481.

[81] Bucks RS, Ashworth DL, Wilcock GK, Siegfried K. Assessment of activities of daily living in dementia: development of the Bristol activities of daily living scale. Age Ageing 1996; 25(2): 113–20.

[82] Juva K, Mäkelä M, Erkinjuntti T, et al. Functional assessment scales in detecting dementia. Age Ageing 1997; 26(5): 393–400.

[83] Thom D. Variation in estimates of urinary incontinence prevalence in the community: effects of differences in definition, population characteristics, and study type. J Am Geriatr Soc 1998; 46(4): 473–80.

[84] Whitehead WE, Borrud L, Goode PS, et al. Fecal incontinence in US adults: epidemiology and risk factors. Gastroenterology 2009; 137(2): 512–7.

[85] Young J, Hood C, Gandesha A, Souza R. Royal College of Psychiatrists (2013). National Audit of Dementia care in general hospitals 2012–13: Second round audit report and update. Editors: London: HQIP. Available at: http://www.rcpsych.ac.uk/pdf/NAD%20NATIONAL%20REPORT%202013%20reports%20page.pdf. Accessed April 24, 2016.

[86] Elia M. Screening for Malnutrition: A Multidisciplinary Responsibility. Development and Use of the Malnutrition Universal Screening Tool (MUST) for Adults. Malnutrition Advisory Group (MAG), a Standing Committee of BAPEN. Redditch, Worcs.: BAPEN; 2003.

[87] Riviere S, Gillette-Guyonnet S, Andrieu S, et al. Cognitive function and caregiver burden: predictive factors for eating behaviour disorders in Alzheimer's disease. Int J Geriatr Psychiatry 2002; 17(10): 950–5.

[88] Chalmers J, Pearson A. Oral hygiene care for residents with dementia: a literature review. J Adv Nurs 2005; 52(4): 410–9.

[89] Kayser-Jones J, Bird WF, Paul SM, Long L, Schell ES. An instrument to assess the oral health status of nursing home residents. Gerontologist 1995; 35(6): 814–24.

[90] Chalmers JM, King PL, Spencer AJ, Wright FA, Carter KD. The oral health assessment tool - validity and reliability. Aust Dent J 2005; 50(3): 191–9.

[91] Evans JR, Fletcher AE, Wormald RP, et al. Prevalence of visual impairment in people aged 75 years and older in Britain: results from the MRC trial of assessment and management of older people in the community. Br J Ophthalmol 2002; 86(7): 795–800.

[92] Chronic Conditions: A challenge for the 21st century. National academy on an aging society number 1 November 1999. Available at: http://www.agingsociety.org/agingsociety/pdf/chronic.pdf. Accessed on April 24, 2016.

[93] Lin FR, Metter E, O'Brien RJ, Resnick SM, Zonderman AB, Ferrucci L. Hearing loss and incident dementia. Arch Neurol 2011; 68(2): 214–20.

[94] Allen NH, Burns A, Newton V, et al. The effects of improving hearing in dementia. Age Ageing 2003; 32(2): 189–93.

[95] Achterberg WP, Pieper MJ, van Dalen-Kok AH, et al. Pain management in patients with dementia. Clin Interv Aging 2013; 8: 1471–82.

[96] Kovach CR, Noonan PE, Griffie J, Muchka S, Weissman DE. The assessment of discomfort in dementia protocol. Pain Manag Nurs 2002; 3(1): 16–27.

[97] Netuveli G, Blane D. Quality of life in older ages. Br Med Bull 2008; 85 (1): 113–26.

[98] Levasseur M, St-Cyr Tribble D, Desrosiers J. Meaning of quality of life for older adults: importance of human functioning components. Arch Gerontol Geriatr 2009; 49(2): 91–100.

[99] Addington-Hall J, Kalra L. Measuring quality of life: who should measure quality of life? BMJ 2001; 322: 1417–20.

[100] Taylor A, Gosney MA. Sexuality in older age: essential considerations for healthcare professionals. Age Ageing 2011; 40(5): 538–43.

[101] Acute care toolkit 3: Acute medical care for frail older people March 2012. Available at: https://www.rcplondon.ac.uk/sites/default/files/acute-care-toolkit-3.pdf. Accessed on March 12, 2014

[102] Aithal S, Patel P, Budhihal D, Davies K, Ramakrishna S, Singh I. An association between increasing age and the clinical outcomes of a geriatrician led emergency frailty unit (EFU) in an enhanced local general hospital. British Geriatrics Society 2016 Spring Meeting. Available at: http://www.bgs.org.uk/pdf_cms/admin_archive/2016_spring_abstracts.pdf. Accessed on April 25, 2016

[103] Singh I. Training and professional development for nurses and healthcare support workers: supporting foundation for quality and good practice for care of the acutely Ill older person. Int Arch Nurs Health Care 2015; 1: 007.

[104] Singh I, Morgan K, Belludi G, Verma A, Aithal S. Does nurses' education reduce their work-related stress in the care of older people? J Clin Gerontol Geriatr 2015; 6: 34–7.

[105] Okeke J, Subhan Z, Twine C, Edwards T, Morgan K, Singh I. The impact of a systematic nurse training programme on falls risk assessment and falls incidence: a study based in a 100% single-room elderly care environment. Age Ageing (2015) 44 (2): 10–1.

[106] Bowling A, Kennelly C. Adding quality to quantity: older people's views on quality of life and its enhancement. London: Age Concern; 2003.

[107] Lien WC, Chang JH, Guo NW, Lin YC, Hsieh PC, Kuan TS. Determinants of perceived physical environment barriers among community-dwelling elderly in Taiwan. J Nutr Health Aging 2015; 19(5): 575–82.

[108] Mental Capacity Act 2005 (UK). Code of Practice. Issued by the Lord Chancellor on 23 April 2007 in accordance with sections 42 and 43 of the Act. Available at: http://www.direct.gov.uk/prod_consum_dg/groups/dg_digitalassets/@dg/@en/@disabled/documents/digitalasset/dg_186484.pdf. Accessed on April 24, 2016

[109] Woodard J, Gladman J, Conroy S. Frail older people at the interface. Age Ageing 2010; 39 (1): i36.

[110] Perrels AJ, Fleming J, Zhao J, et al. Place of death and end-of-life transitions experienced by very old people with differing cognitive status: retrospective analysis of a prospective population-based cohort aged 85 and over. Palliat Med 2014; 28(3): 220–33.

[111] Crowther J, Wilson KC, Horton S, Lloyd-Williams M. Palliative care for dementia-time to think again? QJM. 2013; 106(6): 491–4.

[112] McCarthy M, Addington-Hall J, Altmann D. The experience of dying with dementia: a retrospective study. Int J Geriatr Psychiatry 1997; 12(3): 404–9.

[113] Stuck AE, Siu AL, Wieland GD, et al. Comprehensive geriatric assessment: a meta-analysis of controlled trials. Lancet 1993; 342(8878): 1032–36.

[114] Huusko T M, Karppi P, Avikainen V, et al. Randomised, clinically controlled trial of intensive geriatric rehabilitation in patients with hip fracture: subgroup analysis of patients with dementia. BMJ 2000; 321: 1107–11.

[115] Cameron ID, Lyle DM, Quine S. Accelerated rehabilitation after proximal femoral fracture: a randomized controlled trial. Disabil Rehabil 1993; 15(1): 29–34.

[116] Nikolaus T, Specht-Leible N, Bach M, Oster P, Schuerf G. A randomised trial of comprehensive geriatric assessment and home intervention in the care of hospitalised patients. Age Ageing 1999; 28: 543–50

[117] Asplund K, Gustafsen Y, Jacobsson C, et al. Geriatric-based versus general wards for older acute medical patients: a randomised comparison of outcomes and use of resources. J Am Geriatr Soc 2000: 48: 1381–8.

[118] Counsell SR, Holder CM, Liebenauer LL, et al. Effects of a multicomponent intervention on functional outcomes and process of care in hospitalised older patients: a randomized controlled trial of acute care for elders (ACE) in a community hospital. J Am Geriatr Soc 2000; 48: 1572–81.

[119] Ellis G, Langhorne P. Comprehensive geriatric assessment for older hospital patients. Br Med Bull 2005; 71(1): 45–59.

[120] Bachmann S, Finger C, Huss A, et al. Inpatient rehabilitation specifically designed for geriatric patients: systematic review and meta-analysis of randomised controlled trials. BMJ 2010; 340, c1718.

[121] Covinsky KE, King JT Jr, Quinn LM, et al. Do acute care for elders units increase hospital costs? A cost analysis using the hospital perspective. J Am Geriatr Soc 1997; 45(6): 729–34.

[122] Covinsky KE, Palmer RM, Kresevic DM, et al. Improving functional outcomes in older patients: lessons from an acute care for elders unit. Jt Comm J Qual Improv 1998; 24(2): 63–76.

[123] Ellis G, Whitehead MA, Robinson D, O'Neill D, Langhorne P. Comprehensive geriatric assessment for older adults admitted to hospital: meta-analysis of randomised controlled trials. BMJ 2011; 343: d6553.

[124] Singh I, Hubbard RE. Teaching and learning geriatric medicine. Rev Clin Gerontol 2011; 21: 180–92.

[125] Aithal S, Kaur M, Singh I. Does dementia training change attitudes and competence in dementia care among foundation year trainees? A pilot study. Age Ageing 2015; 44 (suppl 2): ii17.

Chapter 4

An Overview of Polypharmacy in Geriatric Patients

Bilge Sözen Şahne

Additional information is available at the end of the chapter

http://dx.doi.org/10.5772/64793

Abstract

Ageing causes a decrease in cognitive and physical abilities, thus making the elderly more sensitive and vulnerable. Besides, the elderly' living conidtions are greatly affected by various diseases and other health-related problems. As is known, a large number of medicines are used to treat the health-related problems in elderly. Multiple drug use can be named as polypharmacy, though many definitions for "polypharmacy" are available in the literature. Many studies are available to explain the situation of the polypharmacy. Furthermore, there are many studies that confirm the prevalence of polypharmacy in several countries such as Brazil, the Netherlands, Sweden and Singapore. Health professionals involve in different stages of the health care services from the prescription until the usage of the drugs. Especially, pharmacists have significant role in informing the patients about rational use of drugs. It is known that the metabolism in geriatric patients changes with ageing. Therefore, medications, particularly polypharmacy, can cause serious side effect in geriatric patients. However, effective communication between the pharmacists and the patient and reasonable intervention by the pharmacist could prevent the negative effects caused by medications. In addition, an ethical perspective is crucial for considering geriatric patients' benefit.

Keywords: polypharmacy, geriatrics, pharmaceutical services, health care services

1. Introduction

Due to technological developments, in the last century, the life expectancy has increased, so the number of old people has been increasing in the world population. Baby boomers, people who were born between 1946 and 1964, are ageing [1].

However, the birthrate has decreased and the demographic structure of the population has changed [2]. Furthermore, the populations in the most developed countries already have aged [3]. For all these reasons, senility has become an important issue [4].

Senility is a special part of the life course, which differs from person to person because of several reasons like genetic factors and lifestyle. In this period, decreased cognitive and physical abilities make this people more sensitive and vulnerable. Besides, various diseases and other health-related problems affect elderly's living conditions and life quality [5–8]. Some of the reasons of these are as follows [9–12]:

- Some changes take place in the gastrointestinal tract.
- The liver function differentiates.
- The amount of body secretions varies.
- The amount of body water decreases.
- Because of all this, changes in absorption and effect of drugs occur.
- Reduction in sensory perception is seen frequently.
- Emotional changes can be intensely seen.

The World Health Organization defines the memory loss, urinary incontinence, depression and falls or immobility as "four giants of geriatrics" [3, 9]. To solving all of these problems, medication treatment comes into prominence. However, the drug response of geriatric patience is changed because of some reasons like [13]:

- Accumulation of drugs which are eliminated by the kidneys
- Increase in drug binding
- Increase in dispersion of fat-soluble drugs
- Decrease in dispersion of water-soluble drugs
- Accumulation of drugs which are metabolized by liver
- Tendency to heart failure
- Variable dosage regimes

The term of "*polypharmacy*" originated from a Greek word "*poly*" which means "more than one" generally [14, 15]. Multiple drug use can be named as polypharmacy, but there are many different definitions for this term in the literature [14, 16–23]. Some of these definitions are listed below:

- *"Medication did not match diagnosis"*
- *"The use of several drugs concurrently for the treatment of one or more coexisting diseases"*
- *"Concurrent use of 5–9 drugs"*

• *"The use of potentially inappropriate medications, which can increase the risk for adverse drug events"*

Besides, according to some definitions, topical and herbal drugs, vitamin and minerals are not included to the polypharmacy. On the other hand, the duration of therapy is important on polypharmacy for some definitions [16].

In this context, one of the most common definitions of polypharmacy is the concurrent use of six or more medications by a patient. The number of medications varies from 4 to 10 in different studies [20, 21, 24–26]. In some researches, 0–4 drug use is named as non-polypharmacy, concurrent use of 5–9 drugs defined as polypharmacy, on the other hand 10 and more drugs as excessive polypharmacy [21].

As is known, a large number of medicines are used to solve the health-related problems encountered in elderly [11, 19, 27, 28]. Also, the elderly can use many non-prescription drugs with prescription drugs [16, 22, 29, 30]. In order to overcome the side effects caused by drugs used in the treatment of certain diseases, additional drugs are used, but it may cause polypharmacy [16].

There are several problems that may be caused of polypharmacy. In general, the reduction of water consumption and the increase in the body's water supply with ageing, and even in some cases starting to use taking medicaments with food instead of water, is one of these problems. Besides, some other problems that may arise can be listed as below [16, 18, 31, 32]:

- Drug-drug interactions,
- Drug-food interactions,
- Adverse drug reactions,
- Compliance problems,
- Increasing emotional problems,
- Various financial problems.

For all this reason, polypharmacy is a particular concern for all community, especially elderly.

2. Polypharmacy practices in the world

It is known that major medication safety concern in elderly patients is polypharmacy and potentially inappropriate medication use [24]. Polypharmacy draws the attention as an increasingly critical problem in the health care systems, especially on the geriatric patients around the world.

Many studies are available to explain the situation of the polypharmacy in the literature. Most of the studies are made in nursing homes where elderly people live in close quarters [20, 21, 28, 33].

According to the results of a longitudinal study made by Veehof et al., polypharmacy is increasing [33]. Furthermore, there are many studies, which confirm the prevalence of polypharmacy from several counties like Brazil, the Netherlands, Sweden and Singapore [16, 18, 20, 24, 28, 31, 34, 35].

There are also some researches about the commonly used drugs for geriatric patients. Some of the most widely used drugs in geriatrics are as follows [13, 24, 34, 35]:

- Proton pump inhibitors
- H2 receptor blockers
- Beta-blockers
- Diuretics
- Statins
- ACE inhibitors
- Non-steroidal anti-inflammatory drugs

Drug-drug interaction is an important problem for polypharmacy in geriatric patients. Some studies are focused to this problem [36, 37].

Some drugs combination like carbamazepine-nifedipine, warfarin-acetic acid derivate, haloperidol-escitalopram, *Ginkgo biloba*-warfarin are defined as "drugs that should not be combined" because of their dangerous interactions [37]. These interactions can be resulted with possible increased bleeding risk or drug concentration problems [37].

In addition to these, the drug interaction risk must be considered during the use of some drugs like cimetidine, sucralfate, ketoconazole, omeprazole, phenobarbital and clomipramine [36].

One of the important studies about polypharmacy in geriatric patient is SHELTER Study from the Europe. This study includes 4156 nursing home residents from seven European Union countries. According to the results of this research, 49.7% of the residents use 5–9 drugs and 24.3% of the residents use 10 or more drugs [21, 38].

In another study, Junius-Walker et al. found that most of the prescription and non-prescription drug consumers are elderly in Germany [32]. The study sample contained 466 geriatric patients and 26.7% of them were on prescribed polypharmacy. When the OTC user was included to them, this ratio increased to 53.6% [32].

Cankara et al. have investigated the polypharmacy presence in a university hospital in Turkey [35]. According to this study, most of the polypharmacy patients were middle aged and elderly. A hospitalized geriatric patient used 340 different active substances during 30 days [35].

In Spain, San-Jose et al. showed that polypharmacy became prevalent in patients and older than the younger elderly [34]. Besides, they stated that potentially inappropriate medicine is associated with polypharmacy during the use of 10 or more drugs [34].

An important result of polypharmacy is drug-related problems. Finkers et al. found that 96% of the geriatric polypharmacy patients in the Netherlands' nursing homes had one or more drug-related problem like decreased renal function and elevated liver enzymes [20]. Polypharmacy is a common practice to treat geriatric patients; also, it was found in 58.59% of the nursing home residents [28].

Like many other countries in the world, polypharmacy is also widespread among geriatric patients in Sweden. Moreover, Haider et al. revealed that there are significant differences in drug use in different educational groups of geriatric patients [24].

3. The role of pharmacists and other health care professionals in polypharmacy

Health professionals involve in different stages of the health care services from the prescription until the usage of the drugs [14, 19]. Geriatric patients are an important part of the patient group on briefing because of their cognitive abilities. Especially, pharmacists as the most easily accessible health professionals have significant role on informing of the patients about rational drug use [4, 27].

Pharmacists show ultimate attention to provide information to the patients [39]. Particularly with the spread of self-treatment efforts, the role of the pharmacists has become more important [40].

Especially geriatric patients use non-prescribed drugs as well as the prescribed drugs [29], and this situation may cause major problems. Old patients, due to their chronic diseases, since they use more drugs than other age groups and they are more likely to be under risk, they are frequently in communication with their pharmacists [41].

In addition to these, there are many reasons of geriatric patients' pharmacy visits [4]:

- Buying prescription and non-prescription drugs,
- Consulting about their health status,
- Getting vaccine injections,
- Learning to use some medical devices,
- Measuring blood pressure,
- Chatting.

In pharmacy selections of the elderly patients, the quality of the services provided by the pharmacy and the pharmacist's characteristics play an important role. It is indicated that geriatric patients prefer responsible, friendly and cooperative pharmacists [41].

In addition, geriatric patients are expecting the pharmacists to give them information like side effects of the medications and drug-drug interactions [19, 27, 31, 41]. During these briefings, asking open-ended questions makes it easier to understand probable problems [8]. Moreover, counselling services that can be provided along with are thus aligned as follows [4]:

- To control the drug interaction
- To listen to the patient with patience
- To counsel according to patient status
- To continue the counselling process until the patient understands

It should be noted the importance that it will provide important benefits to In order for pharmacists to make appropriate interventions about the use of drugs, it is necessary that the pharmacy service is patient oriented and the relationship between the patient and the pharmacist is important [4, 31, 39, 41].

Furthermore, the pharmacist-physician communication is also important to improve patient care [27, 42]. With an appropriate communication between them can prevent possible medication errors. Also, with this collaboration, geriatric patients' drug compliance gets easier.

Pharmacists have to be more careful when taking the geriatric patient's medication history and medication use-misuse choices should be considered. Especially, it is important to be careful about non-prescribed drugs [29].

Among health service providers, pharmacists take an important place and to provide better service, they have to have sufficient information to make appropriate interventions [42]. During their undergraduate educations, the pharmacists must have detailed information about the geriatric patients, and if it is provided, the service they provide will be more qualified [43].

The physicians' poor prescribing practices are also a common reason of the negative effects of polypharmacy [44]. Therefore, physicians' care and attentions have a core importance.

In addition, in the health services provided to the elder people, at common approaches that lead to various problems particularly like polypharmacy, to prevent patient injury, all health personnel should be working as a team.

In necessary cases, while prescribing appropriate drugs, physicians should cooperate with the pharmacists and the nurses while tracking and applying the drugs for the patients who are hospitalized and who are staying in nursing homes should come together with the pharmacists in necessary cases, and this will minimize the problems faced by the use of drug of older patients.

Moreover, at various problems that the patients in question are facing, orienting the patients to the specialists like physiotherapists and dieticians who are experts in their fields will contribute positively to the quality of life of the patients.

4. Salient points on polypharmacy

It is known that many changes take place on geriatric patient's metabolism. Therefore, side effects of medications have negative impact on geriatric patients, particularly polypharmacy.

Pharmacokinetic changes are one of the most common reasons of polypharmacy's harmful effects on geriatric patients. Some of these changes are listed below [45–48]:

- Absorption problems can be occurring because of the high gastric pH, insufficient absorption space and gastrointestinal motility. Because of these, solubility and chemical stability of drugs can be changed and active transport can be decreased. In addition to these, the risk of esophageal lesions can be increased.
- The composition of body and the permeability of blood-brain barrier can be changed. Moreover, protein-binding sites can be reduced. These changes affect the distribution of drugs, for example, changes on the volume of distribution for lipo-soluble drugs and water-soluble drugs.
- Decrease on the activity of cytochrome P450 and hepatic blood flow affect the metabolism.
- Excretion also changes because of the decreased rate of glomerular filtration and tubular secretion. These cause problems on the elimination of water-soluble drugs.

However, an effective communication between the pharmacists and the patient and reasonable intervention by the pharmacist could prevent these negative effects [19, 25, 27].

Some of the important points that the other health personnel with the pharmacists should pay attention in the application of polypharmacy for the geriatric patients are listed as below:

- While informing the patients with vision loss occurring by senility, caution should be exercised. In cases where written information should be given, attention should be paid to the preparation of the articles can be read easily.
- Especially in some regions, it should not be forgotten that some geriatric patients' reading level is low. In those types of cases, especially while preparing reminders regarding when and how to use the drugs, it would be useful to use pictograms.
- Hearing loss is common in geriatric patients is a condition that should not be forgotten during providing health services. Especially while informing those patients, it is necessary to set the voice tone appropriately.
- It would be helpful to use special drug cases for easy tracking especially for the patients who have memorial problems like dementia. If necessary, the related health personnel should come into play while placing the pills to the boxes that will be used daily, weekly and monthly.
- It should be considered that the geriatric patients' physical strength may be decreased and especially the drug packages, which are developed to protect the children, should be packed by using different packages for the elderly.

Also, an ethical perspective is crucial for considering geriatric patients' benefit. Like in the other patient groups, for the provision of the pharmacy services by especially paying attention to the secrecy of the geriatric patients, there must be a separate place in pharmacies to protect privacy [40].

Besides, in some cases, dementia has caused some problems with regard to informed consent and autonomy, which are important ethical component. Therefore, attention should be paid to taking geriatric patients' history and informing them. Health care professionals must be more careful especially during the polypharmacy.

Also, the principle of justice should not be forgotten during the allocation of limited health resources [49]. It is known that there is no clear solution for these kinds of ethical dilemmas [50]. However, the vulnerability of the geriatric patients should be always considered and health care professionals should give particular importance their beneficence and autonomy [51]. With all that, the principle of non-maleficence must be considered using the evidence-based treatments for geriatric patients [52].

In conclusion, to decrease negativity that may be originated from polypharmacy, the cooperation of the health personnel and the patient relatives is of great importance. Together with adopting and generalizing rationalist drug use, reaching the requested treatment results, increasing the life quality of patients and decreasing the costs would be possible.

Acknowledgements

The author would like to thank Prof. Dr. Selen Yeğenoğlu from Hacettepe University Faculty of Pharmacy for her valuable contributions and support.

Author details

Bilge Sözen Şahne

Address all correspondence to: bilgesozen@yahoo.com

Hacettepe University Faculty of Pharmacy, Department of Pharmacy Management, Hacettepe University, Ankara, Turkey

References

[1] Zagaria MAE. Caring for the aging: key health care legislation. US Pharm. 2009;34(6): 22-4.

[2] Gülhan R. Rational drug use in elderly. Okmeydanı Tıp Dergisi. 2013;29(2):99-105.

[3] United Nations, Department of Economic and Social Affairs, Population Division (2013). World Population Ageing 2013. ST/ESA/SER.A/348.

[4] Yeğenoğlu S, Baydar T. Information and observations of community pharmacists on geriatric patients: a qualitative study in Ankara City. Turkish Journal of Geriatrics. 2011;14(4):34-351.

[5] Vidyadhar TVV, Sushma M, Mohanraj R, Babu M. Polypharmacy in geriatrics. PharmaTutor. 2014;2(5):179-84.

[6] Fulton MM, Riley AE. Polypharmacy in the elderly: a literature review. Journal of the American Academy of Nurse Practitioners. 2005;17(4):123-32.

[7] Gürcü S, Baydar T. Yaslılarda Bilinçli ve Güvenli İlaç Kullanımı [Safe and Rational Drug Use in Elderly]. In: Kutsal YG, editor. Sağlığımız Önceliğimizdir [Our Health is Our Priority]. Ankara: GEBAM; 2013.

[8] Pelicano-Romano J, Neves MR, Amado A, Cavaco AM. Do community pharmacists actively engage elderly patients in the dialogue? Results from pharmaceutical care consultations. Health Expectations. 2015;18(5):1721-34.

[9] Gökçe Kutsal Y, editor. [Aging World and Aging Human]; 2012: Algı Publisihing.

[10] Özer E, Özdemir L. Rational drug usage in elderly and nurse's responsibilities. Nursing Journal. 2009:42-51.

[11] Gökçe Kutsal Y. Polypharmacy in elderly. Turkish Journal of Geriatrics. 2006:37-44.

[12] Ouslander JG. Drug prescribing for the elderly. Western Journal of Medicine. 1981;135(6):455.

[13] Kirilmaz B. Interactions and side effects of cardiovascular drugs in the elderly. Turkish Journal of Geriatrics. 2010;2:107-113.

[14] Bushardt RL, Massey EB, Simpson TW, Ariail JC, Simpson KN. Polypharmacy: misleading, but manageable. Clinical Interventions in Aging. 2008;3(2):383.

[15] Maher RL, Hanlon J, Hajjar ER. Clinical consequences of polypharmacy in elderly. Expert Opinion on Drug Safety. 2014;13(1):57-65.

[16] Medeiros-Souza P, Santos-Neto LLd, Kusano LTE, Pereira MG. Diagnosis and control of polypharmacy in the elderly. Revista de Saúde Pública. 2007;41(6):1049-53.

[17] Patterson SM, Hughes C, Kerse N, Cardwell CR, Bradley MC. Interventions to improve the appropriate use of polypharmacy for older people. The Cochrane Library. 2012.

[18] Lees J, Chan A. Polypharmacy in elderly patients with cancer: clinical implications and management. The Lancet Oncology. 2011;12(13):1249-57.

[19] Takane AK, Balignasay M-D, Nigg CR. Polypharmacy reviews among elderly populations project: assessing needs in patient-provider communication. Hawai'i Journal of Medicine and Public Health. 2013;72(1):15.

[20] Finkers F, Maring JG, Boersma F, Taxis K. A study of medication reviews to identify drug-related problems of polypharmacy patients in the Dutch nursing home setting. Journal of clinical pharmacy and therapeutics. 2007;32(5):469-76.

[21] Onder G, Liperoti R, Fialova D, Topinkova E, Tosato M, Danese P, et al. Polypharmacy in nursing home in Europe: results from the SHELTER study. The Journals of Gerontology Series A: Biological Sciences and Medical Sciences. 2012;67(6):698-704.

[22] Maggiore RJ, Gross CP, Hurria A. Polypharmacy in older adults with cancer. The Oncologist. 2010;15(5):507-22.

[23] Viktil KK, Blix HS, Moger TA, Reikvam A. Polypharmacy as commonly defined is an indicator of limited value in the assessment of drug-related problems. British Journal of Clinical Pharmacology. 2007;63(2):187-95.

[24] Haider SI, Johnell K, Weitoft GR, Thorslund M, Fastbom J. The influence of educational level on polypharmacy and inappropriate drug use: a register-based study of more than 600,000 older people. Journal of the American Geriatrics Society. 2009;57(1):62-9.

[25] Turhan Ö, Kibar E, Ekren E, Engin O, Ercan D, Erdal AI, et al. Medication adherence in elderly: a university hospital-based and descriptive study. Nobel Medicus. 2014;10(2):31-8.

[26] Ziere G, Dieleman JP, Hofman A, Pols HA, Van Der Cammen TJM, Stricker BH. Polypharmacy and falls in the middle age and elderly population. British Journal of Clinical Pharmacology. 2006;61(2):218-23.

[27] Keshishian F, Colodny N, Boone RT. Physician-patient and pharmacist-patient communication: geriatrics' perceptions and opinions. Patient Education and Counseling. 2008;71(2):265-84.

[28] Mamun K, Lien CTC, Goh-Tan CYE, Ang WS. Polypharmacy and inappropriate medication use in Singapore nursing homes. Annals of the Academy of Medicine Singapore. 2004;33(1):49-52.

[29] Stone JA, Lester CA, Aboneh EA, Phelan CH, Welch LL, Chui MA. A preliminary examination of over the counter medication misuse rates in older adults. Research in Social and Administrative Pharmacy. 2016; doi: 10.1016/j.sapharm.2016.01.004.

[30] Michocki RJ, Lamy PP, Hooper FJ, Richardson JP. Drug prescribing for the elderly. Archives of Family Medicine. 1993;2(4):441.

[31] Rollason V, Vogt N. Reduction of polypharmacy in the elderly. Drugs and Aging. 2003;20(11):817-32.

[32] Junius-Walker U, Theile G, Hummers-Pradier E. Prevalence and predictors of polypharmacy among older primary care patients in Germany. Family Practice. 2007;24(1):14-9.

[33] Veehof L, Stewart R, Haaijer-Ruskamp F, Jong BM. The development of polypharmacy: a longitudinal study. Family Practice. 2000;17(3):261-7.

[34] San-Jose A, Agusti A, Vidal X, Formiga F, Gomez-Hernandez M, Garcia J, et al. Inappropriate prescribing to the oldest old patients admitted to hospital: prevalence, most frequently used medicines, and associated factors. BMC Geriatrics. 2015;15:42.

[35] Cankara FN, Asçı H, Sönmez Y. Physcians' drug preferences and polypharmacy presence in inpatients of university hospital. SDÜ Sağlık Bilimleri Dergisi. 2015;6(1): 20-5.

[36] Nawaz R, Hayat S, Khursheed A, Yusuf R, Majeed I. Study of drug-drug interactions in polypharmacy. Indo American Journal of Pharmaceutical Research. 2015;5(4):1563-9.

[37] Oesterhus R, Aarsland D, Soennesyn H, Rongve A, Selbaek G, Kjosavik SR. Potentially inappropriate medications and drug-drug interactions in home–dwelling people with mild dementia. International Journal of Geriatric Psychiatry. 2016; doi:10.1002/gps.4456

[38] Vetrano DL, Tosato M, Colloca G, Topinkova E, Fialova D, Gindin J, et al. Polypharmacy in nursing home residents with severe cognitive impairment: results from the SHELTER Study. Alzheimer's & Dementia. 2013;9(5):587-93.

[39] Salter C, Holland R, Harvey I, Henwood K. "I haven't even phoned my doctor yet." The advice giving role of the pharmacist during consultations for medication review with patients aged 80 or more: qualitative discourse analysis. BMJ. 2007; 334(7603):1101.

[40] Veiga P, Lapao LV, Cavaco AM, Guerreiro MP. Quality supply of nonprescription medicines in Portuguese community pharmacy: an exploratory case study. Research in Social and Administrative Pharmacy. 2015;11:880-90.

[41] Shiyanbola OO, Mott DA, Croes KD. The structural and process aspects of pharmacy quality: older adults' perceptions. International Journal of Clinical Pharmacy. 2016;38:96-106.

[42] Tarn DM, Paterniti DA, Wenger NS, Williams BR, Chewing BA. Older patient, physician and pharmacist perspectives about community pharmacists' roles. International Journal of Pharmacy Practice. 2012;20(5):285-93.

[43] Divine HS, Cain J. Simulation project in a geriatrics course in a college of pharmacy. JAGS. 2009;57:1487-91.

[44] Montamat SC, Cusack B. Overcoming problems with polypharmacy and drug misuse in the elderly. Clinics in Geriatric Medicine. 1992;8(1):143-58.

[45] Corsonello A, Abbatecola AM, Fusco S, Luciani F, Marino A, Catalano S, et al. The impact of drug interactions and polypharmacy on antimicrobial therapy in the elderly. Clinical Microbiology and Infection. 2015;21(1):20-6.

[46] Nobili A, Garattini S, Mannucci PM. Multiple diseases and polypharmacy in the elderly: challenges for the internist of the third millennium. Journal of Comorbidity. 2011;1(1):28-44.

[47] Vestal RF. Pharmacology and aging. Journal of the American Geriatrics Society. 1982;30(3):191-200.

[48] Hammerlein A, Derendorf H, Lowenthal DT. Pharmacokinetic and pharmacodynamic changes in the elderly: clinical implications. Clinical Pharmacokinetics. 1998;35(1):49-64.

[49] Sözen Sahne B, Sar S. Ethical evaluation of the pharmacy services for geriatric patients. In: İlkılıç İ, Ertin H, Brömer R, Zeeb H, editors. Health, Culture and the Human Body – Epidemiology, Ethics and History of Medicine, Perspectives from Turkey and Central Europe. İstanbul: BETİM Center Press; 2014.

[50] Leibovici L, Paul M. Ethical dilemmas in antibiotic treatment: focus on the elderly. Clinical Microbiology and Infection. 2015;21(1):27-9.

[51] Wolf R. General medical and ethical problems of drug treatment in the elderly. Therapie. 1996;51(4):424-8.

[52] Le Couteur DG, Ford GA, McLachlan AJ. Evidence, ethics and medication management in older people. Journal of Pharmacy Practice and Research. 2010;40(2):148-52.

Chapter 5

Role of LTACH in Chronic Critical Illness in the Elderly

Thiruvoipati Nanda Kumar

Additional information is available at the end of the chapter

http://dx.doi.org/10.5772/64865

Abstract

Long-term acute care hospitals (LTACH) have become an integral part of the health care continuum since they were established in the USA in 1999. Many elderly patients admitted to intensive care units (ICUs) survive an acute episode of illness but do not recover fully and develop chronic critical illness (CCI). These patients have been stabilized in short-term acute care hospitals with completion of diagnostic workup and transferred to LTACHs. Elderly patients who have CCI form an important group of patients admitted to LTACHs. LTACHs are organized to provide multidisciplinary management that includes complex medical therapies such as ventilator weaning and dialysis, intravenous therapies like total parental nutrition, complex wound care and rehabilitative services, including physical, occupational and speech therapies. Consistent with high disease burden of comorbidities and poor outcome in the subset of patients with CCI, palliative care should become an essential component of the post-acute care continuum (PACC). LTACHs play a pivotal role in transitioning these patients across the PACC. Details regarding the organization of LTACHs, management of patients with special reference to CCI and perspectives for future advances are discussed in this chapter.

Keywords: long-term acute care hospital (LTACH), chronic critical illness (CCI), post-acute care continuum (PACC), elderly, ventilator, outcomes

1. Introduction

Advances in medicine and intensive care have led to many elderly patients surviving acute phase of illness, leading to a state of chronic critical illness (CCI) requiring specialized treatments for a prolonged period of time [1–3]. Since their creation in the USA in 1999, long-term acute care hospitals (LTACHs) have become an integral part of the post-acute health care continuum (PACC), serving medically complex patients for a period initially envisaged as more than 25 days [1, 4]. While LTACHs typically admitted patients who were difficult to wean from mechanical ventilation, they now cater to a wider range of patients with complex medical conditions in the setting of chronic comorbidities like congestive heart failure, end-stage renal disease, diabetes mellitus type II and chronic difficult to heal wounds. Elderly patients with chronic critical illness are an important and challenging subset of patients admitted to the long-term acute care hospitals, after stabilization in intensive care units (ICUs) in short-term acute care hospitals (STACH) [5].

Chronic critical illness is a devastating condition resulting many times from respiratory failure with difficulty to liberate from mechanical ventilation and characterized by prolonged debility, multi-organ dysfunction, physical and cognitive impairments [2]. A course complicated by intercurrent illnesses, poor outcomes, and high mortality is a hallmark of chronic critical illness in the elderly. LTACHs are organized to provide such multidisciplinary specialized care. Being the first destination in post-acute care, long-term acute care hospitals play an important role in defining the aggressiveness and level of care and arranging appropriate transition of care, as these patients still remain with significant comorbidities and cognitive and functional impairments.

This chapter deals with details regarding the organization of LTACHs and management of chronic critically ill patients, including incorporation of palliative care approaches. Defining aggressiveness of care, directives regarding cardio-pulmonary resuscitation and discharge disposition to the next level of care are addressed. These issues will need further refinement as advances in medicine including pharmaco-therapeutics, genomic health and outcomes research enhance our understanding that can be incorporated into our decision making.

2. LTACH: organization and services

Patients admitted to acute hospitals and intensive care units suffer a wide variety of acute severe illnesses such as sepsis, respiratory failure with sepsis, pneumonia, chronic obstructive pulmonary disease (COPD), cardiac, neurological, hepatic, renal, gastrointestinal, oncological illnesses, trauma, post-operative states, etc. While they survive the acute phase, recovery is incomplete, and they require complex specialized inpatient management for prolonged period of time. About 10% of patients with acute respiratory failure become chronically critically ill [5]. LTACHs have come to be established to provide such level of specialized multidisciplinary care at a cost lower than that of intensive care units. Coordination of expertise specially geared to treat such patients with complex comorbidities is accomplished by a multidisciplinary team. Patients requiring weaning from prolonged mechanical ventilation and those with conditions requiring inpatient care for about 25 days are usually admitted to the LTACHs. Among the elderly population, many suffer from acute illnesses including sepsis, severe pneumonia, endocarditis, vascular events, post-operative complications, trauma in the setting of chronic disease burden such as congestive heart failure (CHF), COPD, end-stage renal disease (ESRD) on dialysis, immunocompromised states, malnutrition, neurological and musculoskeletal impairments. These patients have completed diagnostic workup and require comprehensive medical management that may include mechanical ventilation, dialysis, intravenous therapies for antibiotics, total parental nutrition, complex wound care management including excisional debridement, and rehabilitative services including physical, occupational therapies. They do not, however, require the level of monitoring and diagnostic services available in intensive care units, and can be provided at a lower cost in LTACHs.

High-intensity monitoring and treatment targeted at their acute illness and decompensation with meticulous attention to other chronic illnesses is required to lead to improved outcomes in terms of medical management and improvements in functional capacity. LTACHs provide an opportunity to discharge patients at an early stage from intensive care units [6]. While the need for 25 days of stay was a main determinant for LTACH admissions in the past, experience gained so far in terms of quality of care, outcomes and cost are leading to refinements in the patient selection criteria.

There are two types of locations for long-term acute care hospitals. Some are freestanding, separate hospitals while others operate as a specialized unit within the hospital called "hospital in hospital" set-up. Freestanding hospitals are developed to provide a full gamut of services and multidisciplinary coordination. They have enough bed strength to support provision of those services. Hospital within hospital units provide benefits in facilitating early transition to the next level of care while having the advantage of acute hospital ancillary services and other consultative services at the doorstep. Short-term acute hospital operations are benefited by freeing of ICU beds, better utilization of the available space by leasing to LTACHs and providing ancillary diagnostic services [7].

2.1. Criteria for LTACH admissions

The majority of LTACH admissions are Medicare beneficiaries. The following criteria have to be met for admission to LTACHs: Patients must be screened prior to admission regarding their appropriateness for admission to LTACH in terms of their medical complexity and requirement of inpatient services for a longer period and should be validated within 48 hours of admission [1, 6].

- **(a)** Daily physician visits and review of progress with availability of necessary consulting physicians at the bedside on a timely basis.
- **(b)** Regular review and evaluation of the need for continued care in the LTACH with appropriate discharge disposition if the patient does not meet criteria for care in LTACH.
- **(c)** An individual treatment plan must be formulated for each patient by the interdisciplinary health care team including physicians.
- **(d)** An average length of stay more than 25 days was required for all Medicare patients. There is a welcome shift in emphasizing the need for complexity of medical care with a multidisciplinary team approach rather than adherence to 25-day length of stay as the main criteria. Adjustments in financial reimbursements will however follow.

As the criteria for requirement of average length of stay undergoes revision, financial reimbursements may be impacted. But greater number of medically complex patients that would benefit from the intensity of care and multidisciplinary approach offered in LTACHs could be cared for and have better outcomes. The heterogeneity of patient population and the smaller number of patients admitted to LTACHs make it difficult to study the outcomes comprehensively. But continued attention to quality metrics and refinements is essential. The quality metrics measured and reported include ventilator weaning, wound healing and prevention of pressure ulcers, avoidance of STACH readmissions, catheter-related blood stream infections, mortality and patient safety indicators [7].

As the treatment progresses in LTACHs, the interdisciplinary team plays an important role in consolidating the progress materialized and charting a course for further transition to home or appropriate venue of care, establishing future advance directives on appropriate level of care and coordination of post-acute services. The above characteristics of LTACHs and the delineation of services provided make them an obvious venue for treating chronic critically ill elderly patients who survive catastrophic severe illnesses.

3. Chronic critical illness

While advances in critical care have resulted in improved survival from acute illness, it has led to a large group of patients who are chronically critically ill.

These patients have difficulty weaning from mechanical ventilation, require high-intensity therapeutic, rehabilitative services, and suffer from chronic debility and cognitive and physical decline punctuated by intercurrent illnesses. The number of these patients is increasing and constitutes about 10% of patients with respiratory failure admitted to intensive care units with mechanical ventilation. Protracted recovery period and poor outcomes are a hallmark of this group. More than 50% of such patients are above 65 years. There is a 50% mortality at the end of first year and only 10% are living at home at the end of one year, albeit with some impairment [2, 4, 5]. The incidence of chronic critical illness has doubled with each decade consistent with the increase of aging population and availability of critical care services. The overall annual health care cost of chronic critical illness has exceeded 20 billion dollars in the United States and is steadily increasing [2, 6].

The clinical phenotype is easily recognizable at the bedside by the constellation of clinical features and context. But the heterogeneity of clinical conditions that lead to chronic critical illness as well as varied presentations render difficulties in arriving at a precise clinical definition.

3.1. Defining features of chronic critical illness

While a strict definition is elusive, patients considered to have the syndrome of chronic critical illness in various studies have included [2, 4–6]:

(1) Respiratory criteria in the setting of

(2) Chronic pathophysiological state

http://dx.doi.org/10.5772/64865

(1) Respiratory criteria:

(a) Respiratory failure with a difficulty to wean requiring prolonged mechanical ventilation for at least 21 consecutive days for at least 6 hours a day. Patients requiring mechanical ventilation for at least 96 hours and an ICU length of stay for at least 21 days.

(b) Patients with mechanical ventilation for at least 96 hours with a tracheostomy placement when done for a condition other than head, neck or face disease. Tracheostomy placement indicates a clinical judgment that patient survived from acute episode with no impending signs of death but unable to liberate from mechanical ventilation. Tracheostomy placement is considered a turning point in the progression of course from acute to chronic critical illness [3, 5].

(c) Patients who required at least ten days of mechanical ventilation and not expected to die or be liberated from mechanical ventilation in the next 72 hours were also considered to have chronic critical illness in some studies.

(d) Patients with respiratory failure transferred to LTACHs are generally considered to have entered the stage of chronic critical illness, as the initial purpose of creation of LTACHs was to serve patients that require prolonged services.

(2) Chronic pathophysiological state:

The patients that progress to chronic critical illness form a variety of conditions have a chronic pathophysiological state with persistent inflammation that seems to diminish the physiological reserves and impairs repair [2, 4, 8]. It comprises elements of multi-organ dysfunction encompassing various systems as follows:

- Cardiac
- Renal
- Hepatic
- Endocrinopathy with hormonal dysregulation including loss of pulsatile anterior pituitary hormone secretion, stress hyperglycemia,
- Severe functional decline associated with axonal neuropathy
- Decreased muscle mass with increased adiposity
- Anasarca with hypoproteinemia
- Increased susceptibility to infections and sepsis with resistant organisms
- Encephalopathy manifesting as varying degrees of delirium and cognitive impairment
- Wounds escalated by immobilization including nutritional deficiency, incontinence, infection.
- Malnutrition

3.2. Limitations in the use of respiratory failure in defining chronic critical illness

(a) Patients who are medically complex requiring prolonged medical management share pathophysiological features characteristic of chronic critical illness but do not need intubation with mechanical ventilation or tracheostomy. Examples of such patients include those with severe COPD and respiratory failure requiring high flow oxygen and non-invasive ventilation for prolonged periods, patients requiring longer term inotropes, left ventricular assist devices, and those elderly patients with sepsis and chronic comorbidities [5]. This group includes patients who survived medical or surgical illness that did not require mechanical ventilation but required prolonged inpatient care and form a significant population of patients admitted to LTACHs. These patients are considered to have chronic critical illness.

(b) Patients requiring mechanical ventilation for neuro-degenerative disorders or myopathic conditions without the comorbid burden pathognomonic of chronic critical illness. Examples are amyotrophic lateral sclerosis and muscular dystrophies. Such patients do not share the pathophysiological substrate and are not considered to have chronic critical illness.

4. Clinical features: course and outcomes of chronic critical illness

The clinical picture of elderly patient with chronic critical illness is characterized by recovery from acute critical illness with ventilator dependence, debility, delirium, severe functional decline, in the setting of multiple comorbidities and immunocompromised states. Accordingly, they have ongoing complex medical therapies continued from short-term acute hospitals or intensive care units that include mechanical ventilation, dialysis, intravenous therapies for antibiotics or total parental nutrition or complex wound care. The course is complicated by infections, sepsis and intercurrent illnesses involving other organ systems. While many patients are unable to express their symptoms due to their physical and mental conditions, they suffer from significant symptoms both physical and psychological. These include pain, dyspnea, anxiety, unsatisfied hunger and thirst. The other signs and symptoms are related to the precipitating acute illness, preexisting comorbidities, intercurrent illness and complications during the course of treatment [3]. Hence, they encompass multiple organ systems and vary from patient to patient due to the heterogeneity of these conditions [3, 9]. Following is a list of conditions involving patients with chronic critical illness:

- Respiratory: complications associated with ventilation, decannulation, atelectasis, pneumonia, acute COPD exacerbation.
- Cardiac: CHF, cardiomyopathy, cardiac arrhythmias, acute coronary syndromes.
- Renal: acute kidney injury, chronic kidney disease, complications of dialysis.
- Neuromuscular: axonal polyneuropathy, myopathy.

- Neuropsychological: delirium, restlessness, anxiety, psychomotor agitation, post-traumatic stress disorder.
- Gastrointestinal: hemorrhage, ileus, diarrhea, complications of parenteral and enteral nutrition, *Clostridium difficile colitis*.
- Infections: pneumonia, bacteremia without definite source, catheter-related blood stream infections, gram-negative infections, methicillin-resistant staphylococcal aureus, vancomycin-resistant enterococci and other multi-drug-resistant organisms. *C. difficile colitis*.
- Metabolic/nutritional: malnutrition, anasarca, decreased lean body mass, increased adiposity, stress hyperglycemia, hypothalamic pituitary adrenal hormonal dysregulation, increased bone resorption, vitamin D deficiency and electrolyte imbalance [4].

The above-mentioned conditions require strict attention in terms of management and prevention. However, improving the general condition, well-being and emotional state of the patient by diligent attention to nutrition, exercise and mobility, fluid electrolyte balance, emotional support, sleep and avoidance of drug side effects and toxicities should be the corner stone of management of these patients [2, 10].

5. Clinical course and outcome

Consistent with the complexity and multiplicity of problems involved with the care of chronically critically ill elderly patients, the course is complicated by heavy symptom burden, poor outcomes and extensive resource utilization. About 10% of patients who require mechanical ventilation in the ICUs become chronically critically ill. While generalizations of outcome are difficult due to the heterogeneity of patient conditions and features of different venues, about 30–50% are weaned from mechanical ventilation [2]. The duration of time taken for ventilator liberation varies depending on the diagnosis and condition of patients from 16 to 37 days [2]. Patients who cannot be weaned in 60 days are unlikely to wean. A significant number of patients with chronic critical illness successfully weaned from ventilator continue to have poor prognosis and are burdened by comorbid conditions with multi-organ dysfunction, intercurrent illnesses, immunocompromised states with poor functional status and cognitive impairment. There is a high risk of death in three months and 50% of patients are dead by the end of one year. Only 10% of patients are living at home after one year [3, 11].

Elderly patients with multi-organ dysfunction in general have poor prognosis [12]. It is not age alone, but advancing age with comorbidities and limitations in functional status adversely affect survival and prognosis.

Pro Vent score was developed as a prognostic model to predict mortality. Four factors are taken into consideration: (1) age above 50 years, (2) platelet count less than 150,000 microliters, (3) need for vasopressors and (4) need for dialysis are calculated on the twenty first day of mechanical ventilation. The presence of all four factors was associated with 100% mortality at one year [4, 5, 13]. The absence of all four factors was associated with 80% survival at one year.

Physical and cognitive impairments are severe in chronically critically ill in elderly compared to acute phase. Understanding outcomes, modulating treatment and decisions regarding aggressiveness of care should focus not only on mortality but also on effects on functional status and quality of life.

5.1. Venues of care: LTACH and beyond

LTACHs have been in existence since 1999 to serve the needs of medically complex patients that require prolonged hospitalization [6]. Patients requiring liberation from mechanical ventilation constituted an important group of patients admitted to LTACHs. Patients are transferred from short-term acute hospitals to provide care adapted to the special needs of chronically critically ill patients at a low-cost environment [6]. STACHs were able to discharge patients to LTACHs earlier. This enables STACHs to utilize ICU beds for other patients who are in need for acute critical care illness. In LTACHs, results are often optimized in an environment of multidisciplinary approach geared to treat this group of patients with lower levels of monitoring and cost [14]. LTACHs are not uniformly distributed in different states within the USA, and there is a geographical conglomeration in some states while absence of LTACHS in other areas [4, 5, 7]. Such patients are treated by extended length of stay in the ICUs and transferred to other venues in due course. At the end of optimizing treatment based on cardiopulmonary and functional status, patients are discharged to lower levels of care. Depending on their care requirements, they are discharged to home with adequate care giver support and home health services, assisted living facilities, skilled nursing facilities and inpatient rehabilitation facilities. The majority of these patients were living at home prior to their acute critical illness that culminated in chronic critical illness [3]. Patients and families have to grapple with complexities of adapting to a completely different discharge disposition. Movement to and fro between different venues of acute and post-acute care is an important feature in chronically critically ill elderly [4]. Costs of health care are increasing, estimated to have crossed 20 billion annually, while the number of patients with chronic critical illness is also increasing.

5.2. Decision making including aspects of palliative care

Physicians and members of health care team should have a clear understanding and knowledge of outcomes. Attempts to understand patient wishes and preferences regarding cardiopulmonary resuscitation and lifesaving therapies should be made earlier in the course [3]. Symptom relief and palliative care should play an important role [4]. Understanding and explaining principles of palliative care to families are important to root out the misconception that palliative care is giving up. It is striving for the best quality of life appropriate to the condition with full understanding of the risks and benefits involved in chosen therapies. Physicians and members of the health care team should be knowledgeable and recognize that chronic critical illness is a separate pathophysiological entity with different clinical connotations and outcome compared to acute phase of illness. This highlights the need to chart a different course in CCI compared to those with acute critical illness [4]. Individual therapeutic decisions should however align with the patient's overall wishes and goals. Education of health care providers is of paramount importance in improving understanding and decision making by patients and family members who carry a heavy burden [15]. Families need information regarding estimates of survival, functional impairments and needs of care giving. In the proportion of patients who only survive to suffer and die over several months, early institution of do not resuscitate status and palliative measures are meaningful if consistent with patient's wishes.

6. Perspectives for the future

Measures to improve better understanding and treatment of acute critical illnesses like sepsis, acute respiratory distress syndrome and acute kidney injury will decrease chronic critical illness [8].

Improvements in antibiotic stewardship, prevention of nosocomial infections, catheter-associated blood stream infections and new therapies now under investigational phase for *C. difficile colitis* will all play an important role.

Knowledge of chronic critical illness is not widely apparent among the spectrum of health care providers. With increasing aging population, availability and utilization of critical care services worldwide, chronic critical illness should become part of curriculum in medical education [11]. Knowledge of palliative care and adequate deployment where needed should be encouraged.

Although LTACHs are established in the USA, the experiences and perspectives gained in LTACHs could be adapted to suit different locations worldwide.

Genetic studies hold further promise in being able to understand longevity, susceptibility and therapeutic response to certain infections and diseases that may be heritable [16, 17]. Individuals may have targeted therapies appropriate to their genetic studies. Identification of specific biochemical markers in chronic critical illness may play a role in stratification of patients with chronic critical illness.

Increased use of non-invasive ventilation at early stages to prevent endotracheal intubation may decrease complications and the number of patients progressing to chronic critical illness. Improvements to non-invasive ventilation like delivery via helmet interface may enhance tolerability, compliance and effectiveness with diminished air leak.

Acknowledgements

The author gratefully acknowledges the help received from Vibra Hospital of Northern California for the insights gained in the management of LTACH patients, Dr Edward Zawada for sharing experiences regarding CCI from a long, enlightened career, Ms Debbie Monroe (Dignity Hospital) for help with literature search and Dr Simrann Birk for assisting in the preparation of this manuscript.

Author details

Thiruvoipati Nanda Kumar

Address all correspondence to: nanadakumar.th@gmail.com

Vibra Hospital of Northern California, University of California at Davis, Redding, CA, USA

Family Practice Residency Program, Dignity Health, Redding, CA, USA

References

[1] Medicare Payment Advisory Commission (MEDPAC), Report to the Congress Washington D.C: New Approaches in Medicare, Chapter 5: Defining Long Term Care Hospitals 2004;125–134

[2] Nelson JE, Cox CE, Hope AA, Carson SS. Chronic Critical Illness. AM J Respir Critical Care Med 2010; 182(4): 446–454

[3] Nelson JE, Meir DE, Litke A, Natale MA, Siegel RE, Morrison RS. The Symptom and Burden of Chronic Critical Illness. Crit Care Med 2004; 32(7): 1527–1534.

[4] MacIntyre NR. Chronic Critical Illness: The Growing Challenge to Health Care. Respir Care 2012; 57(6): 1021–1027

[5] Carson SS. Definitions and Epidemiology of the Chronically Critically Ill. Respiratory Care 2012; 57(6): 848–858

[6] Donahoe MP. Current Venues of Care and Related Costs for the Chronically Critical Ill. Respir Care 2012; 57(6): 867–888

[7] Grippi MA, Soisson MJ. Long Term Acute Care in the Spectrum of Medicine. The Intensive Care Manual, 2nd Edition, Elsevier Expert Consult - Online and Print. By Paul N. Lanken, MD, Scott Manaker, MD, PhD, Benjamin A. Kohl, MD, FCCM and C. William Hanson, III, MD. 2014, 1088p ; 109: 968–972, ISBN: 978-1-41

[8] Gotts, JE, Matthay MA. Sepsis: Pathophysiology and Clinical Management. British Medical Journal 2016; 353: i1585 doi:10.1136/bmji1585

[9] Estenssoro E, Reina R, Canales H, Saenz MG, Gonzalez FE, Aprea, MM, Laffaire E, Gola V, Dubin A. The Distinct Clinical Profile of Chronically Critically Ill Patients: A Cohort Study. Crit Care 2006; 10: R89 doi: 10.1186/cc4941

[10] Girard K, Raffin TA. The Chronically Critically Ill: To Save or Let Die? Respir Care 1985; 30(5): 339–347

[11] Lamas D. Chronic Critical Illness. The New England Journal of Medicine 2014; 370(2): 175–177

[12] Somme D, Maillet JM, Gisselbrecht, M. Novara A. Ract, C. Fagon, J. Critically Ill Old and the Oldest-Old Patients in Intensive Care: Short and Long Term Outcomes. Intensive Care Med 2003; 29: 2137–2143 doi: 10.1007/s00134-003-1929-2

[13] Carson SS, Kahn JM, Hough CL, Seeley EJ, White DB, Douglas IS, et al. A Multicenter Mortality Predication Model for Patients Receiving Prolonged Mechanical Ventilation. Crit Care Med 2012; 40(4): 1171–1176

[14] Jeremy M. Khan, MD MS, Rachel M. Werner MD PhD, Guy David, PhD, TenHave, PhD, Nicole M Benson, BS, David A. Asch, MD, MBA. Effectiveness of Long Term Acute Care Hospitalization in Elderly Patients with Chronic Critical Illness. Med Care 2013; 51(1): 4–10. doi: 10.1097/MLR.0b013e31826528a7

[15] Carson SS, Cox CE, Wallenstein S, Hanson LC, Danis M, Tulsky JA, Chai E, Nelson JE. Effect of Palliative Care Led Meetings for Families of Patients with Chronic Critical Illness. Journal of the American Medical Association. 2016; 316(1): 51–62. doi: 10.1001/jama.2016.8474

[16] Wood KA, Ely EW. What Does It Mean to be Critically Ill and Elderly? Curr Opin Crit Care Med 2003, 9:316–320

[17] Patel BK, Wolfe KS, Pohlman AS, Hall JB, Kress JP. Effect of Noninvasive Ventilation Delivered by Helmet vs Face Mask on the Rate of Endotracheal Intubation in Patients with Acute Respiratory Distress Syndrome. Journal of the American Medical Association. 2016; 315(22): 2435–2441. doi: 10.1001/jama.2016.6338

Chapter 6

Ethics of ICU Care for the Elderly

Bruce Bartlow

Additional information is available at the end of the chapter

http://dx.doi.org/10.5772/64053

Abstract

Elders being treated in the intensive care units (ICU) require attention to their special needs, problems, and desires. We can use the five principles of Ethics to identify and respect their wishes, while minimizing our harm to their bodies, spirits, and families. Our technology must be adjusted to clear, attainable goals and consideration of the life they are likely to have after the ICU.

Keywords: hybrid femtosecond lasers, ultrahigh intensities, Photochemically driven laser media, Femtosecond system, Laser-matter interaction

1. Introduction

Elders who find themselves suddenly admitted to a critical care unit may deserve special consideration as we make our ethical decisions. As adults become more dependent on their children, role reversals and projections from an earlier time may muddle the picture of who is the decision maker, who is being cared for and who burdened, and the economics of societal responsibility.

How do we apply traditional ethical principles to this unique group? Is the last of a long time on this planet just a series of losses and wasted resources, or one blessed chance to complete a lifetime of beginnings? How can we help patients and families navigate through the late chapters of this irreversibly terminal process – life?

1.1. "It takes a lot of gold"

A few years after completing my fellowship in nephrology, I realized I wanted to be a pediatric nephrologist. Striding into Children's Hospital, Oakland, CA, I announced my intention.

The response was consistent and clear: "These children are not just little adults. They are their own beings. If you want to pursue that path, you can start over at internship". And that was the end of that.

Decades of adult Critical Care and Nephrology later, I'm well on my way to becoming an Elder – or maybe just old. As I contemplate what might be unique in ethical management of the elderly subjected to Critical Care, I'm surprised at the contradictions in my view of who "they" are. Are the elderly just adults grown grumpy and a bit battered, or a special subset of the disabled? Should they be covered by the Americans with Disability Act (ADA)? Like children, are they unable to represent themselves, instead being under the care and control of those who used to be their children? Or are they uniquely valuable vessels of experience and wisdom who deserve our most tender protection? Are they a drag on our economy, or the only real history we have?

Do the few months to years they have left make investing in them a terrible waste? Or does a lifetime of connection, labor, procreation and contribution to society make every remaining minute worth saving? How should I and society balance saving a few weeks or years of sometimes difficult, potentially limited life against the decades we might have saved by pouring those resources into a young person? Are all years of life of equal value? And whose value system will decide?

Walking home up the hill from my hospital in San Francisco, one of my patients could usually be found resting on his front stoop. "Enjoying your Golden Years?" I'd call out. He'd grunt and reply, "Yeah, they're Golden alright. Takes a lot of gold to get through 'em". I realize now he wasn't just talking about insurance copays and costs of medicine, the struggle to get to a doctor's office, the pharmacy, the lab and home without falling and breaking a hip. It was a toll metered out in aches, pains, serial losses, suffering, fear, constant decisions about how far to push; fighting, hoping; and eventually letting go, searching for the right way and time to say goodbye. It wasn't just about this one superannuated adult. It was the systole and eventual diastole of a heart deep in the chest of a family and a community.

1.2. To be or not to be: that is not the question

Critical care practice is the pursuit of how much can be done. Ethics asks the question, what *should* be done, and which *goals* are worthwhile.

St Luke's Hospital established San Francisco's first Subacute Unit, a place for patients in probably permanent coma or ventilator dependence. As families arrived with their loved one, I'd ask, "Is this how your family member would want to spend the remaining months or years of his or her life?" The answer was almost always, "Absolutely not".

Why, then were we doing this?

Typically the response was, "Because one day the doctors came to us and asked, did we want them to keep doing everything, or let Dad die? We couldn't bear being responsible for deciding to give up" (**Figure 1**) [1].

http://dx.doi.org/10.5772/64053

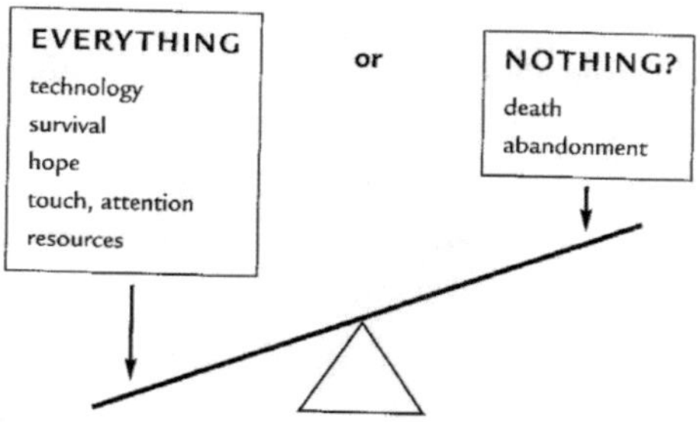

Figure 1. Everything or nothing (Medical Care of the Soul).

Twenty percent of Americans will die in the ICU, accounting for much of the 25% of all Medicare expenditures consumed in the last year of life [2]. Of those in ICU, half will be over 65 years of age. Twenty-five percent of ICU patients over 70 will not leave ICU, compared to roughly 8% of those less than 70. Of the elderly who do survive ICU, many will have experienced significant decline in cognitive or physical function [3–5]. Reported mortality rates vary from 38% at 3 months to 50–80% at a year after ICU [6–9]. Pre-hospital functional status adds additional risk: functionally limited patients experienced higher in-hospital mortality (32 vs. 16%) than those who were more robust [10]. Barely half of patients over 80 years of age who required mechanical ventilation and pressors survived the hospital stay [11].

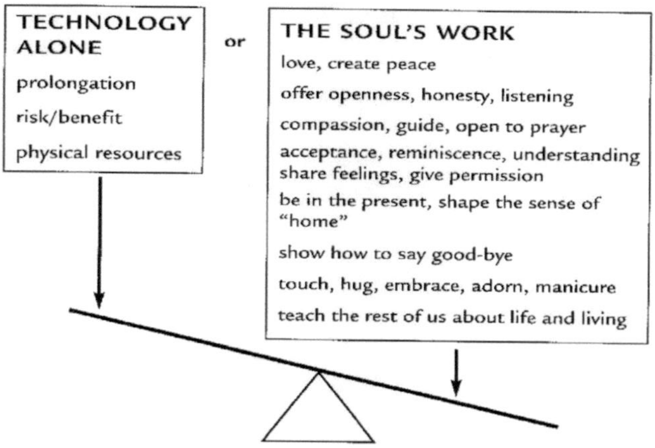

Figure 2. Alternative goals.

I offer these statistics neither to disparage our hubris nor to brag about our successes. Rather, we need to consider what are the goals of our treatment, what burden will be borne and by whom. I learned to ask families and patients a different question: "Faced with a serious or life-threatening illness, would you want us to focus solely on technologic interventions to prolong life, no matter how harrowing? What other meaningful help could we give you in this difficult time?" Some of their answers are in **Figure 2** [1].

1.3. Is age per se a disability under the Americans with Disability Act?

Now, understand, I'm in California. Out here, everybody is disabled and deserves at least two "service animals" to make it through the day; alcoholism, drug abuse, halitosis and the jitters are disabilities; if you don't have a marijuana prescription, you mustn't realize how wrecked you are, and that lack of awareness is its own disability. Folks out here yearn for disabilities, sue for them, and sustain an army of well-healed lawyers to demand them.

The ADA instructs us that the "disabled" are really just "other-abled" and that their limitations must not be considered in our decisions unless – unless – those "other-enablements" make the burden of therapy so intolerable and the benefits of therapy of so little value to the individual that it's cruel to impose the proposed therapy upon them.

Well, we cleared that up, didn't we now?

In my experience, most elderly will fight to the death to be as able as possible. We treat them as disabled at our own risk and should do all possible to support that competency.

Let them have their puppies, their weird hats and habits and their memories. Tailor our therapies to what we presume they can handle. The only disability may be our lack of empathy. And in exactly which textbook, roadside chapel, or CME course are we to find that empathy? The best we can do is an intellectual construct called "Ethics".

Ethics traditionally stands on five pillars: Autonomy, beneficence, non-maleficence, guidance, and distributive justice (aka husbanding society's resources) (**Figure 3**). I would add a sixth: shaping a story, a legacy, that will ennoble the last of this singular life.

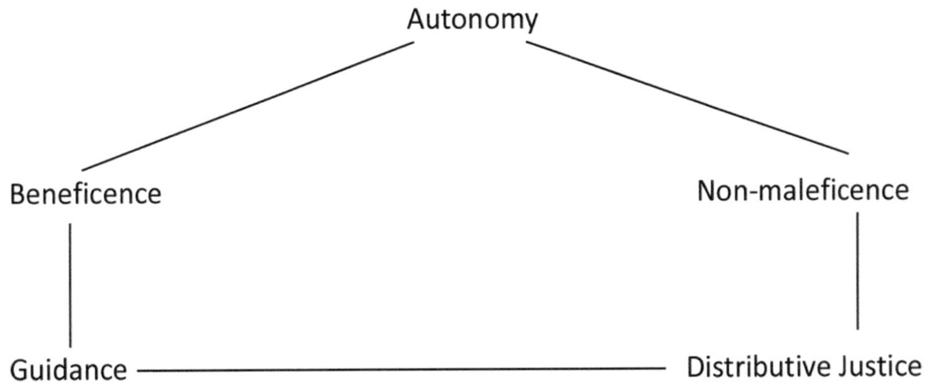

Figure 3. The ethical pentagram.

2. Autonomy

Autonomy is best defined as "the right to refuse unwanted touching". Many cultures or societies consider individual rights subservient to the imprimatur of family, tribe, community,

http://dx.doi.org/10.5772/64053

or state. American and in general Western views put individual autonomy at the top of the ethical pyramid, with the individual the decision maker. Confounding issues particularly in the elderly include:

- Questions of the patient's competency.
- Intrinsic unclarity of the Advance Directive (AD)
- Children's and other family members' competing claims to surrogacy and understanding of the patient's wishes
- Misunderstanding of the surrogate as "demander" of services, the surrogate's versus the patient's wishes, and secondary gain that may invalidate the designated surrogate
- Conflicting desires in a patient overwhelmed with the onslaught of technology
- Unrealistic predictions on the part of staff, patients, and family. (This will be discussed under "Guidance".)

2.1. Questions of the patient's competence

Families and staff may dramatically over- or under-estimate the extent to which an elder can make a reasoned decision. A decent guideline in the face of "impaired mental capacity" is, "Can this individual understand the consequences of his or her refusal?" We may fall back on a careful mental assessment or psychiatric evaluation to answer this question. Depression, anger, obstinance, dementia, bewilderment, linguistics, and a fear of offending family or healthcare providers (their lifeline) all may cloudy the soup.

Thankfully, exploration of friends' and family members' remembrance of the patient's prior wishes may support or give pause about the patient's statements. In this regard, elderly are particularly susceptible to spacial/time disorientation, "sundowning", sleep deprivation, drug effects (especially benzodiazepines, sedation, narcotics), hypothermia, hypoxia, or CO_2 retention. Infections, endocrine disorders or acute illness, family coaching or staff persuasion can run riot on one's decision-making capability. Contrariwise, either our reluctance to be "paternalistic" or a subliminal desire to shape their choices to our or our hospital's advantage may induce us to abandon them to uninformed decision making.

Elders may be overwhelmed by the flood of too many or inappropriate choices ("Do you want us to do this or that?", "We can go three different ways here. Which do you choose?", "Do you wish Resuscitation (CPR)?" in a patient who would not benefit from it). Financial issues ("I don't want my family to lose everything I've built") and the wish to continue taking care of loved ones beyond the time of one's ability to do so are ever-present weights. We must minimize these effects – confine the family to input that reassures the patient, and ourselves to questions that don't add to the patient's distress and confusion.

2.2. Intrinsic unclarity of the Advance Directive (AD)

Many AD's spell out what appears to be a DNR as follows:

"I do not wish life sustaining measures if (a) the burden outweighs the likely benefit, (b) I have irreversible coma, or (c) it will only delay my death".

When patients sign this, very few of them or their surrogates realize that: (a) They have no idea what burdens (risk, suffering) are headed their way, nor have they begun to consider what amount of damage would be acceptable for what outcome (benefit, quality of life); (b) irreversible coma usually takes weeks to months to predict; and (c) every breath we take delays our death. At precisely what point do we conclude those breaths are no longer in our best interest?

2.3. Children's and other family members' competing claims to surrogacy and understanding of the patient's wishes

Very few designated surrogates have really explored the elder's quality of life issues, their desires for the last of life, their fears and wishes for what they want to leave behind. Much less would they explore their own motivations. The other family members are even more adrift without a paddle about their role, responsibilities, and rights. Families implode over these issues: "How could you want Mom to die?" "How could you want her to suffer?" Without clear guidance from medical, counseling, and chaplaincy personnel, the resultant wound in a family can suppurate for generations.

Adult children may also believe that their surrogacy begins even when the patient is competent and able to express their wishes, or that it gives them the power to represent their own wishes rather than those of their elder. Not so.

I begin end of life (EOL) discussions, "I'm not asking you to decide if your mother/father lives or dies. Their illness will decide. I'm asking you to tell me what they would be saying if they could: how much they would want me to put them through to attain what quality of life, and what scene they would want at the end. Then I can tell you what I can achieve. If the best I can do is a death they would have hoped for, I'll tell you how we can get there". After they get over the shock that it's not their, but their parent's choice, almost uniformly they appreciate having the burden lifted. I would put this not under paternalism or "maleficence" below but guidance and my sixth pillar.

2.4. Misunderstanding of the surrogate as "demander" of services, the surrogate's versus the patient's wishes, and secondary gain that may invalidate the designated surrogate

How many times we hear, "We have to do everything because that's what Dad said he wanted" [12, 13]. Yet rare is the masochist who would include in their wishes procedures that would be unduly painful or pointless. Patients don't want suffering without a prospect of return to "worthwhile" life. That "worth" must be explored with each individual. For one it may be "Only if I will be independent and not confined to a facility" (hospital, SNF, subacute). For another, "Only if I won't be a burden to my family" (financial? time? distraction from their responsibilities to the grandchildren? watching me deteriorate?). Or another, "As long as I can play bridge and put on my makeup". As long as I don't smell bad".

And we must consider whether the designated surrogate remains valid. Is the IHSS money they receive each month affecting their assessment that Mom would want to be kept alive

http://dx.doi.org/10.5772/64053

though in a condition she never would have wanted? Is the cost of time away from work persuading them it's time for comfort care? Are they acting as loving adults? How much of their animus is a resentful or desperately dependent little child trying to get even or make up for past transgressions? This is not judgmental fantasy. I've lived it, seen myself an experienced physician transformed lickety-split into a babbling child, and seen so many families go through it. Perhaps when it's our parents we're all of these, all the time.

2.5. Conflicting desires in a patient overwhelmed with the technologic onslaught

My parents both refused to establish Advance Directives or read my book. "We're going to beat this cancer" was Dad's refrain. As his gurney was wheeled into the ICU he begged over and over, "No machines. Don't make me suffer". He survived several days, half the time ripping off his O_2, half the time thrashing to have it put back on, long enough to squeeze our hands, throw air kisses and tell a last few long-winded, gasping jokes, and say how much he loved us. Then he was gone.

Technology has its own steamroller momentum. One author observes, "Although patients may not want to die in pain or without family, most prefer not to die at all" [2]. What starts as O_2 soon becomes dialysis, a ventilator and then surgery. What begins as a chemistry panel evolves to a series of tests, an unexpected diagnosis the treatment of which has disastrous consequences. My Father often quoted, "When you're up to your ass in alligators, it's hard to remember your original purpose was to drain the swamp". How often we're sinking in a wallow of serial misadventures that have nothing to do with the presenting complaint. Few of us at any age have the clarity, prescience, and courage to say no at just the right time.

The momentum of technology easily runs over the calm voice that asks, "but, why not?" Even when we use Advance Directives and EOL discussions to try to control the steamroller, far too often the message gets lost on the way to the providers [14].

We owe it to our patients and families to empower them and give them realistic choices – not "Do you want us to do everything (and of course it will come out well), or give up (needlessly).

In our choice of sedation, narcotics, psychoactive drugs, tests, and procedures, I believe we must go beyond "informed consent". We need to give our patients and families the tools to make choices not from fear (namely the current Presidential Campaigns) but from reasonable hope and realistic information.

2.6. Denial of the probable outlook on the part of staff, patients, and family

These will be discussed under "Guidance".

3. Beneficence and non-maleficence

It is said the road to Hell is paved with good intentions. It's possible the road to Heaven might be paved with bad intentions, but I doubt it.

So many of our huge ethical conflicts hang on disagreements about what constitutes an intention to do good (beneficence) and what an intention to do evil (maleficence). Hippocrates' proscription that a physician must never intend to cause a patient's death comes from a time when death was natural, we could do little to prevent it, and to cause it intentionally was offering the devil help for which he had little need.

Today we're much more capable of prolonging a patient's life in a fashion horrifying to them and their family. More and more, death comes only when we permit it by withdrawing our machines, our pressors, our one more round of chemotherapy, and our one more even more brutal surgery.

Calling it "second effect", we pretend there's a clear, bright line between our responsibility to provide support and symptom relief, versus Physician-Assisted Suicide. This line is tethered on either shore by the idea that a medication given to relieve suffering may incidentally (surprise, surprise!) hasten death. The charge nurse at my subacute called me late one night. A terminal, comatose, ventilator-dependent patient had been off the vent for 7 days. The staff and family were suffering terribly. He asked, "Can I plug the trach so he can die peacefully?" Was the patient in pain? No. Were there signs of distress? No. Since we have no permission to consider family or staff distress and pain, my answer was: "No".

There is worry that if we're empowered to cause death at will, we'll be on the "slippery slope" of Nazis getting rid of those we consider unworthy – those with disabilities, minorities, too few years left or too expensive to care for. The economically unworthy. The unproductive. The unpleasant. Those unlike ourselves [15, 16]. I would say this is less a slippery slope than a meadow with lots of overgrowth hiding potholes. Oregon and other experiments show that the option of assisted suicide forces caregivers to provide much better palliation, so suicide is not their patient's only option. And it works. A vast majority of Oregon patients die at home. Only one in 500 directly access the option of physician-assisted suicide [17, 18].

Woody Allen said, "I'm not afraid of death, I just don't want to be there when it happens". Our euphemism for treatment focused on quality rather than quantity of life is "Comfort Care". I'm fascinated that hidden in that is a damning admission: much of what we do to patients is "Discomfort Care". I've proposed in ethics committees at several hospitals that all patients are "Comfort Care" unless on admission we order "Discomfort Care".

We act beneficently when we tailor our offerings to the patient's goals, whatever they may be [19]. When we propose to cause discomfort unlikely to achieve an outcome the patient would appreciate, we're acting maleficently. We provide the most beneficent guidance when we reassure a patient and family that their choice to reject a proposed treatment will be met not with rejection or resentment, but support and a commitment to vigorous symptom management.

I believe that the elderly, who have more experience of loss, suffering, and hard choices than the most of us can imagine, especially need that reassurance.

http://dx.doi.org/10.5772/64053

4. Guidance

Several events in the 1960s and 1970s conspired to change our views of authority. These include the revelations about secret carpet bombings of Cambodia, then Watergate, followed by a series of scandals reminding us that those who had power over us might be acting not in our best interests, but in their own; a burgeoning awareness and resentment of the "paternalistic" all-powerful doctor; the beginnings of informed consent and Advance Directives; rapidly evolving technologies for lethal warfare, even as we learned to sustain life beyond the death of one or more organ systems.

I don't believe these developments were unrelated.

Recently, a local high school teacher asked me to discuss with her class Rebecca Skloot's book, "*The Immortal Life of Henrietta Lacks*" [20]. I was stunned to discover that well into the 1980s, malignant HeLa cells were being injected into prisoners to see if they would "take". The Tuskeegee syphilis project was still going, and even today there are no real guidelines for informing patients when their tissues or fluids are going to be used for research or commercial gain. By no one's fault, "Informed consent" remains a nebulous dream, and the rights of those who are powerless are questionable at best.

Still, I believe the recoil away from paternalism has gone far too far. Instead of trusting whatever the doctor says to do, our patients are now given a grocery list of unweighted options while lawyers are drooling just outside the waiting room door. Once we were a profession. We're well along to becoming shopkeepers too busy watching over our shoulders for the health inspector to remember our calling. We now sell to our "clients" or "stakeholders" – who used to be "patients".

Many elderly don't want a lot of falderal and jabber. I've had Hispanic patients listen to my protracted recommendations and explanations, then reach out, palms up, and answer, "Yo me pongo en sus manos". I put myself in your hands. I'm stunned by the stoicism and submission to fate manifested by many seniors. But we fail them if we accept this cloak of power without adapting our guidance to their values and needs.

I have a few recommendations:

- Learn the truth of what we're providing. Consistently, Critical Care doctors and nurses, Nephrologists and I presume other specialties overestimate the likelihood of successful outcomes at three times what is true. To an ICU nurse or doctor, "success" may be discharge to the floor. To a hospital nurse, discharge to a skilled nursing facility (SNF) or (God willing) home. To a doctor in training, success may be turfing the patient somewhere, wherever the Discharge Planner orders them to send the patient. All our dialysis patients are living. There's no body count of those who have died. As mentioned earlier, we have little idea if they made it out of hospital, nor how long or how well they'll live. The data are there [4, 5]. We fail our patients and our responsibilities when we deny the realities they'll face after discharge. If we don't know the odds, how will we guide our patients and families?

- This is way beyond mere numbers. Dr. Chris McIntyre of Nottingham, England noticed that patients passing his door on the way to dialysis were laughing, chatting, and upright. Those leaving were silent, sullen, and often in wheelchairs. One 26-year old sent him a note to the effect: "I'm not stupid. I know I need dialysis to live. But if what you're doing makes me feel so bad, mustn't it be hurting me?" His and other attentive nephrologists' exploration of that question is transforming dialysis practice.
- Listen and ask. I can't tell my patients whether I can achieve what they'd value if I haven't found out what that is.
- The old "there are no atheists in the trenches" may well be true. Whatever we or our patients believe, the search for meaning, healing and spiritual growth are pervasive [21–23]. We should attend to these yearnings as vigorously as we treat a fever or an infection.
- Don't offer procedures that won't work or will do more harm than good. It's very healing to begin, "I'm not offering you CPR because it won't work, and will hurt you. Ethically, I can't do that". "I'd discourage choosing ventilation, because it will isolate you from your family if it comes to that, and I don't believe it will lead to your getting out of the hospital. Here's what I'd propose instead". "You say what's most important to you is being in the garden with your family and pets. If we go down the technologic route, I don't believe we can get you there. Instead, here's how we could achieve what you want".
- One of the greatest disillusions of Hospice workers is how many patients are referred to them in the last hours or few days of life. So much good could have been done in the months prior. A patient says, "Oh, I'm not ready for hospice". Translation: "I'm not really dying". How about proposing an organization focused on assuring you the best quality life in the time you have left. Would you reject that? Sacrifice time to hold onto denial? The organization of which I speak is called Hospice. Our local Hospice staff assert they're not in the business of dying. They're in the business of fostering the best remaining life possible.
- We should be much clearer about the risks of "Discomfort Care" and much clearer about the manifold benefits of "Comfort care". Patients circling in critical care are somewhat like battered spouses: abused, wounded, desperate, but afraid to say "no" to their abuser. We have the power to turn that "no" into a "yes" for healing.
- Our elders are getting older, our population more diverse. Our physicians and nurses are being driven out of practice earlier by the flurry of computers, computerized documentation and pathways, bean counters and "core measures". Data show that the numbers of administrators/clerks/middle managers/surveillance personnel in healthcare are increasing logarithmically. The number of doctors and nurses is unchanging or shrinking. Income and educational disparity block access to healthcare jobs for many minority groups. That leaves healthcare providers younger, whiter (or more foreign) and less and less like those we serve. We can't evaporate our prejudices or deny our inability to truly empathize with many of our patients. All we can do is recognize our deficiencies, acknowledge them, and ask our patients to guide us through.

http://dx.doi.org/10.5772/64053

5. Distributive justice

Though this may be the ethical principle on which our self-respect and our health care systems succeed or collapse, it's where we most fail [24, 25]. We talk about the disproportionate cost of sustaining the elderly with high-tech medicine. We wring our hands over thousand dollar pills and million dollar treatments when we can't afford immunizations for children. We feel guilty about America's rather mediocre outcomes in a world where most societies can afford about $2 a day for healthcare. Two decades ago, ethicists estimated the cost that America could afford to "buy" an additional year of life was $100,000. I can't imagine what it would be now.

But whose life? And what quality of life? In the collapse of the World Trade Center, the compensation deemed appropriate for a stock broker's life was pegged at hundreds or thousands of times the worth of a cook's life, or the life of the firemen and police who rushed in to save others, or the soldiers, airmen, and sailors who volunteered to sacrifice their lives to try to protect us from another attack.

Some years ago, Bill Mauer and the Robert Woods Foundation put together a magnificent four-part series, "On Our Own Terms (OOOT)". You can order this, watch it, absorb it. I remember two young Asians acting as surrogate for their uncle who'd had a devastating stroke with no chance of recovery. Their decision was something to the effect, "Our culture cherishes and protects our elders. We do not want our uncle to suffer needlessly. We should stop". At the last minute, a social worker piped up, "But he has 100 days of Medicare SNF benefits!" They turned on a dime (or $200,000.) "Oh, then we would want our uncle to be given every chance". One hundred one days later, as they became financially liable, the uncle was withdrawn from life support, never having regained function or consciousness.

So the government and insurance companies try to sway us by tamping down payment and charging us for every complication. Hospitals watch "opportunity days" like hawks or children sobbing over their last precious penny, while their CEOs are amongst the best paid in the world. Workers have to decide between lowering their insurance co-pay or feeding their kids and sending them to a community college. We bluster about "Oh, well, look at how much we waste on wars, corruption, incompetence in the public sector and greedy bankers who get multi-million dollar bonuses for causing the Great Recession".

Then we all get up, buck up, man up and go back to burning all the technologic resources we can.

We are supposed to be husbanding the 15% of our society's resources that go to healthcare. We fail miserably. So, what resources could we protect, and what remaining wealth could we help our patients and families salvage in a time of loss?

6. A sixth pillar: the final scene

The quantity and quality of additional life we can offer our elderly patients is limited. Nevertheless, the memory of that time will be particularly intense, its significance for good or ill, for healing or harm immense, and its lifespan as close to "immortal" as we know. As with the devolution of a woman named Henrietta Lacks into trillions of HELA cells, our human touch and voice during a serious illness can shape most powerfully the individual's sense of their value to their loved ones and their society, while confirming the survivors' best hopes or worst fears for how they can expect to be treated by the world in which they live.

I'm drawn back to the start of this article, my brief dalliance with pediatric nephrology. Pediatricians have told me they mainly take care of the parents. Elder care may be mainly about the children – those who were created by these elders, who carry the treasures and burdens their elders passed on, and will live to make sense of what it was all about.

This "pillar" is a combination of guidance, beneficence, and non-maleficence. It's my impression that the majority of elders understand the fix they're in. Their main concerns are that they not suffer, not be a burden, and that the family and friends they leave behind will be ok. Most family members, when we scrape away all the internal conflicts and unspoken promises, are desperately afraid they'll do something wrong and pray they'll have protected and honored their parent to the best of their ability. Our actions and words can either empower and support those hopes, or shatter them.

Malidoma Some', an African shaman, wrote, "Why do the dead walk where I come from? They walk because they are still as important to the living as they were before … We must see our dead so that we can truly mourn them, all the way through, without restraint, to release the grief from our hearts once and for all" [26]. In the Good Ol' USA, so many lives slip away in an air controlled hospital room. The body is whisked off to a distant mortuary to be gussied up. The last scene is to a large extent in the hands of healthcare workers. Our training for this? Nada. Our comfort with it: Nil. But like a spiritual credit card, the rewards to be reaped? Priceless.

Alas, when I offer our Family Practice residents the chance to put in a central line or intubate a patient, they're on it like tics on a hound. When I invite them to participate in helping shape the last of a patient's life, the vast majority suddenly have to get to that noon meeting instead.

If you're a hammer, everything looks like a nail. If you've never seen a nail, you're not going to be a very good hammer.

I describe in my book a family tearing up the place one midnight of a months-long hospitalization. They were demanding that Mom be re-intubated for a fourth time, though they knew she had no prospect of surviving. The attending Intensivist had the courage to refuse. Called in for an emergency Ethics consult, I asked did they understand she was dying? Yes. Was this how she'd want the last of her life to go? Their answer: absolutely not.

So then, what would she want? They were clear: She'd want to be in bed with her 2 dogs, that stinky comforter she always loved, playing her horrible honky-tonk music and all of us sitting around laughing and crying about great holidays we'd had together.

We told them we could create that scene. They jumped at it.

The nurses moved everything to a larger room, got the Ativan and fentanyl going. Security snuck her dogs up the back stairway. The night nursing supervisor pretended she was blind

http://dx.doi.org/10.5772/64053

and deaf to what was going on, while hauling heaping trays of goodies up from the kitchen. The tribe arrived and made it all familiar.

When I came in the next morning, the music was indeed rowdy, the comforter indeed well suffused with organic history, and the exhausted crowd were crashed all around her bed, reminiscing with much laughter and tears.

"How's she doing?"

"Doc, she died three hours ago. We just couldn't leave her alone quite yet".

If we don't ask, we won't know. As with any procedure, shaping the last of life has risks and benefits, burdens and outcomes. As with any procedure, we can do it well or badly, or miss it altogether.

I believe we should craft the final scene with as much care as we do our H&P, our list of allergies and diagnoses, our SOAP plan and accursed discharge paperwork. The scene and its meaning to the survivors will live decades beyond anything else we do. How do we proceed?

As emphasized by Hospice, it's not what we DO, but just being present. Truly present.

- Listen, learn, ask, be guided.
- Apply our and the family's resources to create a memory which will enrich us all.
- Reassure the patient that indeed their legacy will be a positive one for those they care about, and describe how we will help make that so. What needs to be healed, what said? What will you regret not doing or saying when you had the chance?
- Don't run away to an imaginary meeting.
- Share our gratitude with the patient and family for opening up to include us in their final scene
- Know this is the "Core Measure" by which we will be most remembered and judged.
- Don't forget.

Author details

Bruce Bartlow

Address all correspondence to: bgbartlow@frontiernet.net

Shasta Regional Medical Center, Redding, CA, USA

UC Davis, Davis, CA, USA

References

Ethics of Elderly in ICU

[1] Bartlow B. *Medical Care of the Soul*. Boulder Colo: Johnson Books, 2000.

[2] Angus DC, Truog RD. Toward better ICU use at the end of life. *JAMA* 2016; 315(3):255.

[3] Ehlenbach WJ et al. Association between acute care and critical illness hospitalization and cognitive function in older adults. *JAMA* 2010; 303(8):763.

[4] Ferrante LE et al. Functional trajectories among older persons before and after critical illness. *JAMA Intern Med* 2015; 175(4):53.

[5] Needham DM et al. Improving long-term outcomes after discharge from intensive care unit: report from a stakeholders' conference. *Crit Care Med* 2012; 40:502.

[6] Carson SS. The epidemiology of critical illness in the elderly. *Crit Care Clin* 2003; 19(4): 605.

[7] Bagshaw SM et al. Association between frailty and short- and long-term outcomes among critically ill patients: a multicenter prospective cohort study. *CMAJ* 2014; 186(2):E95.

[8] Tolle SW et al. Characteristics and proportion of dying Oregonians who personally consider physician-assisted suicide. *J Clin Ethics* 2004; 15(2):111.

[9] Consensus statement of the society of critical care medicine's ethics committee regarding futile and other possibly inadvisable treatments. *Crit Care Med* 1997; 25:887.

[10] Sacanella E et al. Functional status and quality of life 12 months after discharge from a medical ICU in healthy elderly patients: a prospective observational study. *Critical Care* 2011; 15:R105.

[11] Daubin C et al. *Health Qual Life Outcomes* 2011; 9(35):1186.

[12] Huynh TN et al. The frequency and cost of treatment perceived to be futile in critical care. *JAMA* 2013; 173:1887.

[13] Roeland E et al. When open-ended questions don't work: the role of palliative paternalism in difficult medical decisions. *J Palliat Med* 2014; 17:415.

[14] Support Principal Investigators. A controlled trial to improve care for seriously ill hospitalized patients. The study to understand prognoses and preferences for outcomes and risks of treatments (SUPPORT). *JAMA* 1995; 274:1591.

[15] Quill TE et al. Responding to patients requesting physician-assisted death. *JAMA* 2016; 315(3):245.

[16] Yang TY, Curlin FA. Why physicians should oppose assisted suicide. *JAMA* 2016; 315(3): 247.

[17] Tolle SW et al. Characteristics and proportion of dying Oregonians who personally consider physician-assisted suicide. *J Clin Ethics* 2004; 15(2):111.

[18] Onwuteaka-Philipsen BD et al. Trends in end-of-life practices before and after the enactment of the euthanasia law in the Netherlands from 1990 to 2010. *Lancet* 2012; 380(9845):908.

[19] Orsini J et al. Assessing the utility of ICU admissions for Octagenarians. *Aging Clin Exp Res* 2015.

[20] Skloot R. *The Immortal Life of Henrietta Lacks*. New York: Crown Publishing Group, 2010.

[21] Block SD. Perspectives on care at the close of life. Psychological considerations, growth, and transcendence at the end of life: the art of the possible. *JAMA* 2001; 285:2898.

[22] Pargament KI et al. Religious coping methods as predictors of psychological, physical and spiritual outcomes among medically ill elderly patients a two-year longitudinal study. *J Health Psychol* 2004; 9:713.

[23] Laytner A. *Arguing with God: A Jewish Tradition*. Lanham, MD: Rowsan and Littlefield Publishing Inc, 1990.

[24] Breyer F. Health care rationing and distributive justice. In *Perspectives in Moral Science*, 2009:395.

[25] Somé MP. *Of Water and the Spirit: Ritual, Magic, and Initiation in the Life of an African Shaman*. New York: Harper and Row Publishers, 1980.

[26] Fowler RA et al. Sex- and age-based differences in the delivery ad outcomes of critical care. *CMAJ* 2007; 177(12):1513.